Sports Cupping Therapy

*The Essential Guide to Chinese Cupping
Therapy and Its Benefits*

Mary Conrad

ISBN: 1975703588
ISBN-13: 978-1975703585

TABLE OF CONTENTS

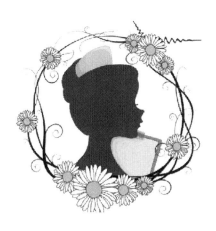

Introduction

Sports cupping therapy is a traditional Chinese therapy that improves the blood flow in the body. It became popular in the West when Michael Phelps was spotted going through this therapy in his latest sportswear commercial.

The cupping therapy is popular amongst sports superstars. A lot of other celebrities such as David Arquete, Jessica Simpson, Victoria Beckham, Gwyneth Paltrow, and Jennifer Aniston are certified cupping fans.

But, what is cupping therapy? What's the science behind it? Why are more and more people hooked up on this alternative medicine?

Cupping therapy is a process of placing bamboo or glass cups on the skin to suck away all the muscle tension and pain. Once the suction begins, the cups are moved across the skin. This technique is known as glide cupping or massage cupping.

Cupping is often combined with acupuncture treatment. But, it has several benefits on its own. Cupping can be used to relieve common issues that athletes face day in and day out. It is used to relieve neck and back pains. It is also used to ease fatigue, anxiety, stiff muscles, migraines, and rheumatism. It can even lessen the appearance of cellulite, releases toxins from the veins, and can increase metabolic processes.

This book will serve as your guide to sports cupping. Here, you'll find everything you need to know about cupping therapy, including:

- ✓ What is sports cupping?
- ✓ The history of sports cupping
- ✓ The science behind sports cupping
- ✓ Acupuncture and cupping
- ✓ How athletes could benefit from cupping therapy
- ✓ Types of cupping therapy
- ✓ List of common sports injuries that can be treated by sports cupping
- ✓ How it works
- ✓ Tools used for sports cupping
- ✓ 389 acupuncture points
- ✓ Cupping Points
- ✓ How it's used for common sports injuries
- ✓ Frequently asked questions about the cupping therapy
- ✓ And more!

This book provides an easy to understand explanation of the cupping therapy, its types, and benefits.

Cupping is not just a fad, it is a therapy that has been used for many centuries. It can do wonders to your sports performance and your overall health.

Take a step towards health and wellness today!

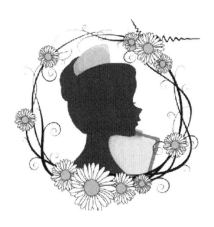

Chapter 1

Sports Cupping 101: What You Need To Know About The Latest Sports Trend

A muscle is like an elastic band. It moves and stretches. Fascia is that layer that surrounds the muscles. If the muscle is attached to the fascia, the muscle is unable to move or stretch. This could restrict movement and it could affect the performance of athletes.

Cupping therapy pulls away the adhesions between the muscle fibers and the fascia to enhance the efficiency of your biomechanics and allow you to move freely and improve your physical performance.

Cupping therapy is a process wherein a trained therapist places a glass, earthenware, silicone, or bamboo cup on the skin to create suction. This suction increases the blood flow and it reduces pain and inflammation.

Cupping therapy is the secret weapon of star athletes like Michael Phelps. Wang Qun, a celebrated Chinese swimmer, proudly showed off her cupping marks during the 2008 Olympics held in Beijing. The players of the New York Mets are also using cupping therapy to improve their performance. But, cupping therapy is not only used by athletes. A lot of other celebrities use cupping therapy to improve their health like Jennifer Aniston, Gwyneth Paltrow, Maria Menounos, Victoria Beckham, David Arquette, and Jessica Simpson.

For those who do not know, cupping therapy is not a new concept. In fact, it has been around for over 2000 years.

History of Cupping

In terms of history, cupping was a technique that was practiced in different parts of the world such as Asia, Africa and Europe. In ancient times, most feared the presence of evil spirits and the possibilities of these spirits causing sickness. African medicine men used to take animal horns, hollow it out and cut off the tips. They used this as a crude but effective method of cupping. Using their mouth, they create suction in the animal horn to treat boils, snake bites and skin lesions. To maintain the suction, they used chewed-up leaves mixed with saliva to plug the hole in the horn.

The written records for cupping date back up to the second century BC. It was mentioned in a book by Bo Shu, written on silk and written during the Han Dynasty. The therapeutic use of cupping was introduced in a book written by Zouhou Fang around 28 AD.

Cupping is extensively used and recorded in China. Around 500 years ago, a Chinese surgeon used this procedure during surgery as a way to divert blood away from the surgical site. Through the years, the practice evolved from the use of crude horns to bamboo, ceramic and glass cups.

Cupping Therapy was also popular in Egypt during the ancient times. In fact, it appeared in an ancient Egyptian text called the Ebers Papyrus. It is one of the oldest medical textbooks. The use of cupping also became popular in Ancient Greece. Hippocrates, the father of modern medicine, used cupping for structural problems and internal disease. He believed that cupping can cure most diseases. Several Greek doctors used cupping to restore the spinal alignment of patients.

Eventually, cupping was used in many countries in Europe and even in South and North America. It was widely used by American and European doctors during the first half of the 18th century. It was used in hospitals and private practices. During this time, a technique called wet cupping or

Hijama became more and more popular in the Middle East. It is a process where the therapist makes small incisions in the patient's skin to dredge the blood, toxins, or poisons out.

By the second half of the 18th century, the popularity of the cupping therapy declined due to the development of a new medical paradigm.

But, in 1950s, China teamed up with the former Soviet Union to conduct an extensive research on the cupping therapy. This research confirmed the clinical efficacy of the cupping technique. Since then, cupping is widely used in government-owned hospitals in China.

In 2004, cupping resurfaced in the west as a celebrity trend when Gwyneth Paltrow proudly showed off her cupping marks at the New York Film Festival. Since then, countless of other celebrities such as Jennifer Aniston, Justin Bieber, Kim Kardashian, and Victoria Beckham followed suit. It was adopted by sport superstars such as Serena Williams.

The cupping therapy became even more popular when swimming superstars sported their cupping marks during the 2016 Rio Olympics. Celebrated Olympian Michael Phelps was also spotted using the cupping therapy for muscle recovery in his Under Armour ad.

Sports cupping is now rising as the new sports trend. In fact, it is recommended by many sports coaches and physical therapists. It is primarily used for muscle recovery.

Cupping and the Qi

Before we discuss how cupping therapy works, let's first discuss the concept of qi. Qi is the most important concept in Traditional Chinese Medicine techniques such as acupuncture and cupping.

Qi is the bioelectric life energy that flows in every human being. It is similar to the concept of prana in ancient Indian medicine. It is the energy that protects the body from external pathogens such as the weather, toxins, bacteria, and viruses. It also cools and warms the body when needed. The qi moves through the energy points in the body called meridians to promote growth and prevent stagnation. If you have good qi, you're energetic and you'll have good endurance. This increases your sports performance.

Having a balanced qi also increases your ability to focus as well as improves your overall health and well-being. When your chi is flowing freely and the opposing forces in your body called yin and yang are balanced, you'll thrive in all parts of your life – health, career, relationships, and personal development.

But, if your qi is not flowing freely in your body, you'll experience fatigue and several other health issues. It can lead to depression and anxiety. This could negatively affect your sports performance. Unbalanced qi also leads to infertility, allergies, liver disease, poor memory, autoimmune disorders, and serious medical disorders. It could hamper the function of your liver, digestive system, brain, lymphatic system, cardiovascular system, and reproductive organs.

There are many factors that hamper the movement of chi in your body, such as stress, anxiety, lack of exercise, and unhealthy diet. Overtraining can also cause qi stagnation.

Cupping therapy treats stagnation and unblocks your qi by increasing the blood flow in your body. It attempts to reinvigorate your body's natural energy flow. It even activates and strengthens your body's self-healing powers.

Cupping in Sports

Cupping has become a new but effective tool in training recovery. It helps by mobilizing the fascia using negative pressure that pulls the skin outwards which is the opposite of how massage is usually done. In massage, the pressure is applied to the skin to reach the muscles beneath. In cupping, the suction helps in moving the stagnant blood as well as loosening the tight muscles and fascia.

Injury in sports is very common. This is especially true for contact sports such as hockey, football and rugby. The body undergoes several processes to naturally heal.

Phases of Healing

The phases of healing first involve an injury. During this critical moment, the body will go through hemostasis. Platelets migrate towards the site of injury and release different chemicals such as cytokines, chemokines as well as hormones.

The blood vessels in the surrounding area constrict to reduce the blood flow to the injury. The exposed skin on the injury site will activate the platelet aggregation which helps the platelets clump together forming a plug and stopping the bleeding. Once the platelets aggregate on collagen, this triggers the platelets to further release chemicals (coagulation cascades) that leads to the first phase of wound healing.

1. INFLAMMATORY PHASE

The clot formation stops. The initial response of vasoconstriction will stop at around 10-15 minutes after the injury. It is then followed by a longer period of vasodilation. The vasodilation allows more blood in the area as well as histamines, prostaglandins, kinins, and leukotrienes. Injured cells are then broken down and macrophages clean up all the debris and bacteria from the injury. This will result in changes to the skin pH, which gives the sensation of pain. Macrophages play a huge role in the entire processes since it releases several chemicals that aid in new tissue formation.

2. PROLIFERATION PHASE

This is the phase where new cells and tissues are formed. It happens in different stages.

Epithelization – This is the stage where the wound is slowly closed over by cell migration to the injury site. This provides the barrier between the wound and the environment.

Fibroplasia – This starts between 3-5 days after the injury and can take up to 14 days to finish. Fibroblast help in the production of collagen, elastin, fibronectin, glycosaminoglycans, and proteases. Inflammation eases and collagen starts connecting the cells together.

Angiogenesis – Blood flow is essential to maintain the growth and health of new cells. New blood vessels are created during this stage if it is necessary. However, unnecessary blood vessels are also discarded via apoptosis.

Contraction – This is a stage where the edges of the wound moves towards the center in an effort to fully close the top and connect the newly formed cells together.

3. MATURATION PHASE

In this phase, the wound undergoes the final stages of healing. Collagen continues to be produced as well as removed when unnecessary. The wound continues to knit together but the new skin will still be less strong when compared to the unwounded area. It could take up to 21 days after the injury before the collagen stabilizes.

When is sports cupping contraindicated?

Cupping in sports injuries is not advised during the ACUTE phase. This is usually the first 48 hours after the injury and is marked with increased blood flow on the injury and inflammation. When there are signs of bleeding (whether internal or external), inflammation, open wounds, fractures and complete tendon ruptures, cupping should not be performed. Skin injuries also don't need cupping therapy since it's often accompanied by open wounds. Before trying out this treatment, it's best to get clearance from your physician.

When is sports cupping advised?

Sports cupping is done during the RECOVERY phase, which is technically the time when physical therapy is advised. It is said to be effective when used to help with muscle recovery and in improving the blood flow to the area.

It is critical to point out that in muscle recovery and healing, blood flow and oxygenation are essential components. Both of which, can be increased and improved with the use of cupping therapy.

How Cupping Works

Cupping is a therapy wherein a therapist heats a glass on the skin to produce suction. Most therapists heat the glass using fire and then places the glass in the affected area. The heat produces a force that sucks out the toxins and lifts the skin. Some therapists use a pump or a vacuum to lift the skin and the muscles.

Cupping therapy draws out old, stagnant, and non-circulating blood and bring them to the surface of the skin, which may leave visible marks. If there's no stagnation in the area, the marks are often very light and would disappear quickly, but if you have an injury, rigid muscles, disease, or if you have a sedentary lifestyle, you'll most likely have dark cupping marks after the therapy. The pattern and color of the marks vary depending on the level of the stagnation in the affected area.

The cupping marks look a bit scary, but the cupping therapy is completely safe when performed by trained professionals.

MARY CONRAD

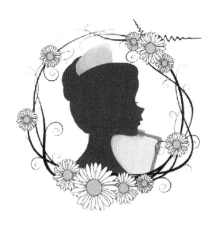

Chapter 2

The Benefits of Cupping

There are many people who are still skeptical of the benefits of cupping. Aside from a study in China in the 1950s, there are several studies conducted to check the effectiveness of cupping in easing muscle pains and improving sports performance.

A research by Hossam Metwally shows that dry and wet cupping techniques are effective in treating myofascial pain syndrome. The study was participated by 42 patients suffering from myofascial pain. These patients were not previously treated using the cupping therapy. Each patient went through cupping therapy twice a week for ten consecutive weeks. The results were amazing. After ten weeks, it was found that all patients noticed improvement and increased mobility. But, patients suffering from neck pain and upper back pain noticed the greatest improvement. A lot of patients continued to use cupping therapy after ten weeks because it made them feel better.

There are about 725 clinical studies conducted on the effectiveness of the cupping therapy from 1958 to 2011 including 419 case series, 30 clinically controlled trials, and 163 randomized controlled trials. These studies show that cupping therapy can reduce the symptoms of herpes zoster, muscle pain, and other diseases.

Cupping therapy has many proven benefits, including:

> **It removes the toxins in the body.**

Eating a lot of over processed food, binge eating, lack of exercise, dehydration, stress, unhealthy diet, and constipation can lead to toxic buildup. When you have too many toxins, you'll often feel tired. You're also prone to weight gain and obesity. Toxic buildup also leads to acne, rashes, muscle pains, bad breath, increased belly fat, lower back pain, breast soreness, low energy, intolerance to fatty foods, diarrhea, flatulence, and lowered resistance to infections.

Sports cupping increases the blood circulation in your body and stimulates the flow of fresh blood.

- This helps flush out all toxins in the body and treat conditions that are associated to toxic buildup such as aches, fevers, allergies, anxiety, poor circulation, muscle pain, coughs, colds, and flu.
- Cupping therapy helps athletes recover from strenuous training. Excessive physical training leads to stress that can result to the toxic build-up in the muscles.

> **It relieves depression and anxiety.**

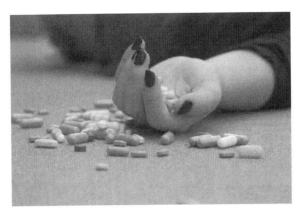

Depression and anxiety can affect individuals of any ages, including sports superstars. Depression can cause daytime fatigue and can affect one's physical performance.

Cupping therapy can reduce the symptoms of depression and anxiety by relaxing and detoxifying the body. It removes the impurities, toxins, dead cells, and other debris from the body. It brings fresh and oxygen-rich blood. Most therapists use a combination of wet cupping and fixed cupping. It usually takes six sessions to alleviate depression and anxiety. Cupping can restore wellness, happiness, and emotional health through restoration of balance in the body.

➤ **It relieves many health conditions.**

If you're a professional athlete, you have to keep your body healthy all the time. Simple health problems such as flu, fever, or bacterial infection can affect your performance.

Cupping can help relieve and prevent many common health conditions such as asthma, common colds, allergies, infections, asthma, irritable bowel syndrome, gastritis, diarrhea, fatigue, abdominal pain, hiccups, acne, high blood pressure, arthritis, migraine, and stomach pain.

Cupping therapy can also cure several more serious diseases such as diabetes mellitus, bronchial asthma, acne, cardiovascular diseases, carpal tunnel syndrome, chest pain, facial palsy, hemorrhoids, hernia, paralysis, cough, anxiety, back pain, depression, shingles, fibromyalgia, and gout. However, some of these claims are not backed by scientific study. For serious illnesses, always consult an expert or a professional in the field.

Most importantly, it alleviates diseases that affect sports performance, such as inflammation, over-training syndrome, exercise-associated muscle cramps, plantar fasciitis, asthma, heat stroke, and rhabdomyolysis.

➢ **It improves sports performance.**

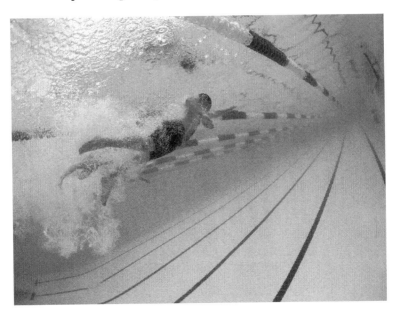

Our bodies have a limit. If you're an athlete, you are often pushing your body to its extent. It can provide rapid muscle relief and eases muscular dysfunction. It improves sports performance in many ways. It loosens tight muscles and adhesions. It literally pulls adhesions apart and it relaxes the tight muscles.

It also improves your sports performance by your increasing blood flow. Poor blood circulation negatively affects your energy and stamina. It can lead to muscle cramps and pain that can limit your mobility and performance. You'll also experience hair loss, varicose veins, lower leg pain, infection, shortness of breath, dizziness, edema, headache, foot ulcers, and changes in skin temperature. Cupping improves blood circulation by pulling the skin into the cup. This draws blood to that area, allowing the blood to flow more freely and speed up the repair of the damaged tissue.

Cupping treats the most common athletic complaints such as plantar fasciitis, muscle spasm, chronic muscle imbalances, joint pain, shoulder pain back pain, and neck pain.

Sports cupping naturally increases stamina and agility. It improves speed, endurance, concentration, and mobility.

> ## It promotes relaxation.

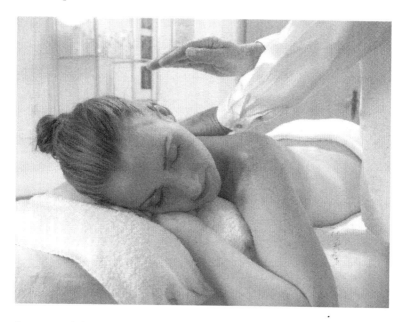

Sports training is stressful - physically and mentally. Stress is more dangerous than you think. It can weaken your immune system and comes with a string of symptoms, including headaches, low energy, loss of sexual desire, chest pain, rapid heartbeat, social isolation, frequent infections, pessimism, and inability to focus. Cupping therapy relieves stress by drawing out the toxins in your body and allowing your energy or qi to flow freely. Cupping balances the distribution of energy and blood in your body, improving the function of your organs and relieving stress.

The cupping therapy is also cost effective and is safe. It does more than improve mobility and increases the elasticity of the muscles. It improves your health and the overall quality of your life as well. It makes you feel more relaxed and gives you the energy to do the things that you wanted to do.

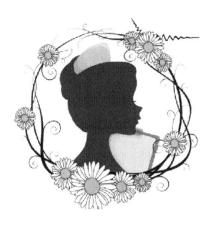

Chapter 3

Types of Cupping Therapy

Cupping has been around for many centuries, so it's no wonder that there are many types of cupping therapy. Each cupping technique is designed to achieve a specific goal. For example, dry cupping primarily releases the adhesions between the fascia and the muscles. The wet cupping technique, on the other hand, is used to draw out toxins.

Dry cupping is primarily used in the West while wet cupping is the technique used in the middle east.

Here's a list of the different cupping therapy types: (this section is fine but it needs fine tuning. Remove the weak, medium and strong cupping and classify it as cupping techniques based on Intensity. Under dry cupping place the vacuum, flash or empty and massage. Under wet, place herbal, water.

Different Forms of Cupping

Dry Cupping

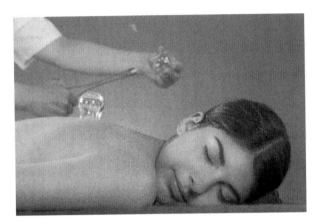

Dry cupping is the most basic cupping technique. This is also called fire cupping. The therapist heats the cup using fire and then quickly places the cup on the patient's skin. The heat sucks and lifts the skin up. The air inside the cup creates a vacuum that reddens and expands the skin. The cup rests on the skin for about 5 to 10 minutes. Most therapists use glass cups for dry cupping because they're more durable and easy to sterilize.

This cupping technique is completely safe and does not cause any pain. You'll simply experience a short pinching sensation. It may take some practice in getting the right amount of heat in the cup when doing fire cupping. A tip is to start off with a small flame and working up from that. For instances when the cups have too much suction and is causing discomfort, press the skin surrounding the cup until air enters the cup. If this fails, lubricate the skin around the cup and move it towards bony areas of the body. This will make it more difficult for the cup to hold the suction and it will pop off.

Wet Cupping

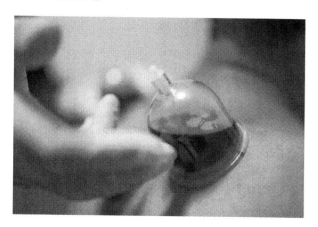

Wet cupping is the most used cupping technique. This cupping type is also known as Hijama and is commonly used in the Middle East. The therapist places a heated cup on the patient's skin and let it sit for about 5 to 10 minutes, allowing the cup to lift the skin up. Then, he removes the cup and uses a blade or a scalpel to make small incisions in the affected area. He then places another cup on top of the incision and uses a pump to draw the toxic blood out and lift the skin up. The therapist then removes the cup and places antibiotic ointments and bandage on the skin to prevent infections.

This cupping technique is definitely bloody and a bit painful. The patient will experience a short pinching sensation because of the incisions. But, there's no need to panic. These incisions heal in a very short time and they do not leave scars. If you have low pain tolerance, you can ask the therapist to use local anesthesia. This technique should not be done at home. Open wounds can lead to infections if the cups aren't sterilized and there are errors in technique.

Massage Cupping

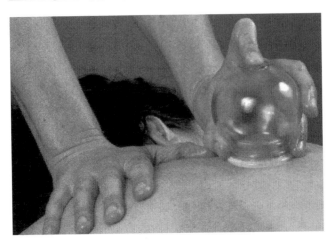

This is a form of dry cupping and it is also known as moving cupping. The therapist applies essential oils on the skin and then places the cup over the affected area or cupping point. Once the suction begins, the therapist moves the cup over the skin. This creates an inverse massage effect – instead of exerting pressure on different massage points of the body for healing, this process uses suction to move the muscles, tissues, and skin upwards. This technique is an effective healing and weight loss tool that's been used by chiropractors, physical therapy, and spa treatment.

Massage cupping improves the blood flow to the muscles and tissues. It softens muscles and loosens knots and adhesions. It also eliminates chronic congestion. This cupping therapy type is so relaxing that the patient may fall into a deep sleep.

Flash Cupping

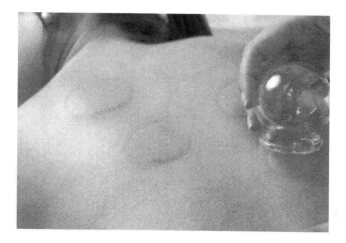

If you want to prefer not to have cupping marks, it's a good idea to choose this technique. Flash cupping is used to apply short interval suction or flashes. The therapist applies healing creams and herbal oils on the skin. He warms the cup using a fire and then places it on the skin for about 5 seconds. He then removes the cup and places it on the skin again for another 5 seconds. This process is repeated many times. This technique is used when cupping the face and other sensitive parts of the body.

It is also a technique that is for the elderly and those with weak Qi. The short intervals help by getting the Qi moving without causing exhaustion to the patient.

Herbal Cupping

This cupping method is used to cure neck pain, shoulder pain, asthma, cough, and common cold. This technique uses various tools such as metal clamps, fire, herbs, water, deep pan, and bamboo cups. The bamboo cups and herbs are placed in a boiling water for about 30 minutes before applying to the skin. The therapist usually uses a wide variety of Chinese herbs such as lotus seed, astralagus, lingzhi or ganoderma, dang gui or angelica sinesis, alisma, ma huang or ephedra sinica, licorice root, gingko biloba, lily bulb, isatis leaf, honeysuckle flower, and perilla leaf.

Water Cupping

This is a complicated process that must only be practiced by highly experienced practitioner. The therapist places ¾ cup of water in the glass and quickly places the cup on the skin without spilling the water. This technique is used to cure asthma, dry coughs, rheumatism, and pain.

Needle Cupping

This is also known as the acupuncture cupping. The needle is applied to the acupuncture points and then, the cup is placed on the site where the needle is located. This technique is used to enhance the effect of acupuncture and can be beneficial for athletes. This technique relieves neck pain, sciatica, stroke, knee pain, biliary colic, headache, hypertension, fasciitis, fibromyalgia, morning sickness, renal colic, rheumatoid arthritis, and allergic rhinitis. This technique also cures a wide variety of diseases such as insomnia, hyperlipaemia, lactation, neurodermatitis, obesity, Raynaud syndrome, reflex sympathetic dystrophy, vascular dementia, urolithiasis, ulcerative colitis, tourette syndrome, sore throat, hepatitis, herpes, female infertility, and osteoarthritis.

Cupping Techniques based on Intensity

- **Weak Cupping:**

Based on its name, this technique offers gentle pressure. The suction is achieved by manipulating the size of the flame or by pulling on the pump gun lightly. It often leaves a light pink circle that often fades within a day.

This cupping method is used to help relax the body and improve blood flow. It helps promote healing by improving the circulation in the body. It can be classified as a light cupping that may be given to patients who are under 7 years old or elderly. The length of the treatment can go as long as 30 minutes. It's recommended for minor health conditions such as colds, asthma, sore throat and tonsillitis.

- ## Medium Cupping:

This technique applies medium pressure or suction. The suction is firm and may feel slightly uncomfortable at first. It will leave visible marks or bruises.

This is the most common technique used for those with strong chi. It is considered safe for children above 7 years to get this particular treatment. The length of the treatment would be 15 minutes. It can be used for headaches, sports injuries and stress-related conditions.

- ## Strong Cupping:

This cupping technique is characterized by a strong suction that often drains the chi. This is often used for detoxification and leaves dark bruises after the treatment. According to Chinese medicine, those bruises are toxins that are removed from the blood and body. This is the type of cupping that is used for chronic musculoskeletal conditions.

Myofascial Decompression Therapy

Myofascial decompression therapy is more commonly known as sports cupping. The traditional Chinese cupping therapy targets the twelve meridians in the body for healing. The myofascial decompression therapy, on the other hand, targets the skeletal and muscular system of the body. Although, several sports cupping therapist uses the acupuncture points. This method usually uses a mechanical vacuum equipment to create suction. The cup is attached to a suction pump and applied to the skin. The therapist usually massages the patient first using cream and herbal oils before placing the cup on the skin.

This cupping technique is used to:
- Decrease myofascial syndromes and faulty patterning due to hypertonic muscles
- Decrease scar adhesions, scar tissue, and myofascial dysfunction
- Decrease the presence of hypersensitive and tender tissues called trigger points

The myofascial decompression therapy is not painful, but it could leave bruises that would disappear after a few days. The reverse pressure exerted by suction increases the flexibility of tissues and relieves swelling. It treats many sports injuries such as workout injuries, tendon injuries, tail bone injuries, muscle soreness, shin splints, rotator cuff tear, groin pull, head injury, concussions, sciatica, ankle injury, Achilles tendon injury, and dislocated shoulder. We will discuss this in detail later on.

Here are a few videos that you might find helpful when trying to find out more on this therapy:

https://www.youtube.com/watch?v=1JpzmdZc2yU
https://www.youtube.com/watch?v=6W2DCLxsT5A

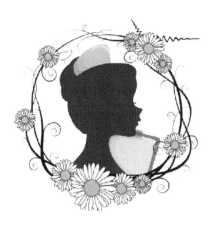

Chapter 4

Who Performs Cupping Therapy?

Cupping therapy is generally safe when practiced by a trained professional. This healing method is usually performed by doctors, chiropractors, acupuncturists, and physical therapists. A lot of sports coaches and massage therapists are also trained to perform this type of therapy.

There are a number of certificate programs and training related to sports cupping and cupping therapy in general, including:

ACE Massage Cupping

This training provides the certification needed to practice massage cupping. As of 2017, this training costs about $140.

The Optimum Cure and Care

This institute is located in the UK, but it offers level 4 courses for therapists from all over the world. You'll receive a diploma and a certificate after completing the course. This certification course costs £650. After completing the course, you can become a member of the General Regulatory Council for Complementary Therapies (GRRCT) and BCS (British Cupping Society).

Hijama Cupping Certification Course

This certification course is designed by the director of the Hijama Clinic and is available for female and male learners. You can complete this training within the day and costs around £475.

Hijama Training Institute

This institute offers an online level 5 higher Diploma Hijama course. It is a course that you can complete in 400 hours, which includes the history of cupping, cupping techniques, and the physiology of the human body. The course also includes a practical training. This training costs around £475.

Contemporary Cupping Methods Certification Program

This training is conducted in different parts of North America, Europe, Canada, and Asia. It includes practical and theoretical training. Trainees get to practice on seven types of cups. The students who complete the training will receive a certification in Contemporary Cupping Therapy. It is a three-day course that costs around $690.

It is important to put your safety first. So, if you decide to undergo this alternative therapy, make sure that it's done by a trained and certified professional.

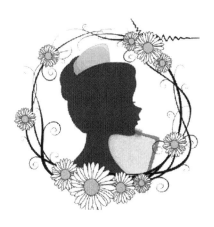

Chapter 5

How To Do Sports Cupping

Sports cupping is the secret weapon of superstar athletes. It looks difficult and overwhelming, but it is relatively easy to do:

Cupping Tools

To get started, you'll need a few tools, including:

<u>Cups</u>

You can use a regular cup, but if you want to get the best out of the treatment, it's best to use special myofascial decompression cups.

Bamboo cups – These cups are used for herbal cupping. These cups are cheap, but you need to polish them using sand paper before using in order to remove the rough edges. The rim of the cup should be smooth. The downside of using bamboo cups is that they are prone to cracking. This leads to air leakages which weakens the suction.

Suction cups – These cups are used in sports cupping and are usually made of plastic. They are break-resistant, convenient, and safe. These cups are usually attached to a pump or a suction device.

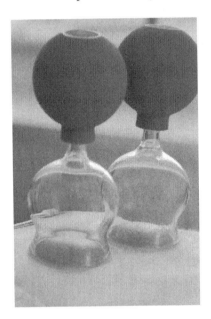

Glass cups – These cups are shaped like a ball. They come in different sizes –medium, small, and large. They are durable and easy to clean.

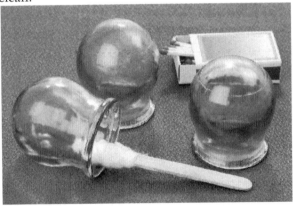

Facial cups – The facial cups are usually small with round pumps.

There are a number of cup sizes, too, including:

Cup Number or Code	Diameter
1	One by six centimeters
2	One by five centimeters
3	One by four centimeters
4	One by three centimeters
5	One by two and ½ centimeters
6	One by two centimeters

You would need at least 6 pieces of cup #1 and then, buy maybe four pieces of cup #2 or cup #3.

Vacuum Suction Pump - There are different types of vacuum suction pumps. The cheapest one is the handheld plastic pump that costs about $0.50. There's also a number of a power press electric pump in the market. It usually costs $38.47.

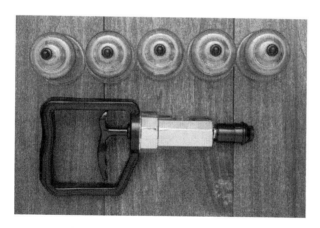

Essential Oils

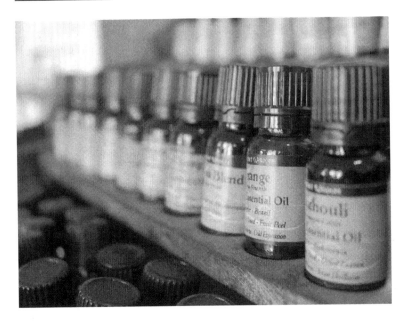

Aromatherapy enhances the effect of sports cupping. To get the best out of cupping, diffuse essential oils such as:

Lavender- This relieves cramps, muscle spasm, rheumatism, and sprains. It also eases stress and anxiety.

Marjoram – This essential oil treat spasms and alleviates stress and anxiety. It is commonly called as the happiness herbs.

Wintergreen – This oil has an anti-inflammatory and anti-spasmodic effect. It is a natural treatment for muscle cramps, muscle spasms, headaches, and muscular pains.

Eucalyptus – This essential oil can do wonders for athletes. It is extremely relaxing and relieves nerve pain and fibrosis.

Peppermint – This oil relieves muscle pain, cramps, and aches. It has strong anti-inflammatory and anti-spasmodic properties.

Clary sage – This essential oil eases respiratory cramps, headaches, and muscle spasms.

Roman chamomile – This is a powerful antispasmodic oil that has strong healing abilities.

Ginger – This essential oil reduces pain and stiffness. It reduces chronic joint pains, tension, tendonitis, and spasms.

Rosemary – This is a relaxing oil that improves the memory. It detoxifies the liver and helps relieve stress.

Ointments - You'd need antibiotic creams to clear the skin and treat blisters. This is especially true when undergoing wet cupping.

Needles

If you're combining acupuncture and cupping, you'll need a set of high quality acupuncture needles.

You can find some of these tools in medical supply stores, but you can also find several high-quality cupping sets in online marketplaces such as eBay and Amazon.

BASIC CUPPING

Step 1
Prepare the cups by washing them using salt water. Make sure that they are clean and dry before using. You should not use the same cup twice. You should use a new set of cups for every patient or have them purchase their own set for their exclusive use. However, if you're using glass cups, these can be sterilized and used again.

Step 2
Determine the patient's complaints and disease by examining the symptoms. Once you identify the disease, you need to identify the

corresponding cupping points of that particular medical condition. For example, if you have neck pain, you have to place the cups on the back, on both sides of the spine.

Step 3
Ask the client to lie face down. To avoid infection, clean the cupping points. Wash the skin with soap and water. Then, apply herbal oil or skin cream.

Step 4
Attach the pump to the cup. Then, place the cup on the skin. Now, press the pump to create suction. Remove the pump, and then place another cup on the skin.

You can use the fire cupping technique if you don't have a pump. Soak a cotton ball in a cup full of pure alcohol. Then, remove the cotton ball from the cup using a pair of forceps and lit the cotton ball using a match. Heat the lid of the glass cups using fire. Then, quickly place the cups on the skin. Check the suction and make sure that it's not too uncomfortable or painful.

Step 5
Once all the cups are in place, there are several ways in going about the treatment. This would differ on the condition of the client. Initially, you can perform static cupping on the sore areas and cupping points. For muscle recovery after workout, you can also perform moving or massage cupping.

Step 6
After 10 minutes, ask the patient to lie face down. Then, remove the cups. Disinfect the blisters or marks using alcohol or an antibiotic ointment.

It takes days before the marks disappear. Cupping therapy for treatment of a muscular condition should be done twice a week for a few weeks. Regularly asses the condition of the muscles before providing the treatment. Once full recovery is received, the sessions can be ceased or decreased as needed.

Massage Cupping

Massage cupping is basically adding movement to the regular cupping practice. The main reason for this form of cupping therapy is to get the lymphatic system moving and the blood flowing. While this is considered a deep-tissue massage, it doesn't require the same amount of effort as a regular massage. When used for post-training or workout recovery, the treatment acts by loosening the fascia and loosening any build-up of fluids in the tissues.

This technique usually uses a single cup at a time and changed according to the body part where you want to do the session.

You'll need:
- Cupping set
- Essential oil or any lotion of choice

1. Ask the client to lie down on a flat surface. It can be massage bed or any comfortable bed that encourages relaxation and is convenient for the procedure.

2. Lightly spread oil on the target area. It's preferable to use therapeutic oils that assists the therapeutic effect. The oil will help by making it easier to move the cups.

3. Prepare the clean cups close to the bed. Usually, only one cup is used at a time but it may vary in size depending on the treatment site.

4. Place the cup on the specific cupping point. If you're using a cupping set with a pump gun and a hose, attach the hose to both the cup and pump gun. This cupping set is more convenient for massage cupping since it's more continuous. When the cup pops off during the massage you can easily pump it up to restore the vacuum. However, you can use any cupping set you have on hand.

5. Create a vacuum using the pump gun to secure the cup. For cupping sets with a vacuum nozzle, just twist it clockwise to

create a vacuum and twist counterclockwise to release.

6. Ensure that the vacuum is comfortable and not painful. Slowly move the cups in an outward motion either away from the center of the body or towards the lower extremities. If you encounter areas where the cup won't move, don't force it. For certified practitioners, these stops are often a signal that there's some congestion in the area and extra work needs to be done for those. The skin in the cup is assessed before proceeding. Continue the massage between 5 to 10 minutes for the first session.

7. Release the suction by pressing right below the rim of the cup for pump gun cupping sets. Massage cupping usually doesn't leave any bruises since it never stays in place for long. However, it may depend on the condition of the client as well as the practitioner who is administering the therapy.

Note: The steps above are quoted from my book titled, *The Basics of Cupping.*

Myofascial Decompression Therapy

Note: Please be reminded that this treatment is better when done by a licensed professional. The main reason is that they have thorough and tested knowledge on the concepts which govern the practice, which is a combination of muscle physiology and the meridians of the body. The steps that are outlined in this section is general and differs according to the site where there was a previous injury or a strained muscle.

What to expect during the treatment?

The provider will assess the symptoms as well as the site of the problem. Range of motion exercises (ROM) will be performed to determine the muscle issues as well as for reference after the treatment. The ROM exercises will be continued throughout the procedure. Patients may be asked to actively flex and extend different muscle groups while the cups are in place

What to expect after the treatment:

Sore muscles and weakness due to active flexion and extension of different muscle groups.

Items Needed:

- ✓ Cupping sets (preferable vacuum cups for easy reattachment and release)
- ✓ Oil or cream

Procedure:

1. Position the client depending on the muscle group targeted.
2. Generously oil the area for better adhesion for the cups. _Optional: The provider may give massage cupping to initially to help relax the patient and the loosen the muscle._
3. Apply the cups along the meridian lines that cross the designated muscle groups or just along the affected muscle

group or scar adhesions.

4. Actively perform range of motion exercises while the cups are attached firmly. This differs according to both the muscle groups and specific sport that the client plays. For runners, the provider could ask them to mimic the muscle movement when their running such as hip flexions and extensions. For swimmers, it might mean a reach and pull movement as if they're swimming.

5. Remove the cups.

6. Asses the areas and compare the previous data with the post-treatment results.

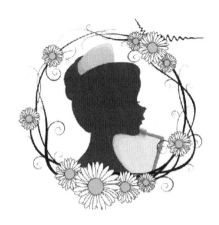

Chapter 6

The Cupping Points

Which part of your body should you cup? The answer is it depends on your medical condition and on the type of cupping therapy that you're using. There are different cupping points in the body as illustrated in the photo below. Each point cures specific diseases.

TIBB CUPPING POINTS

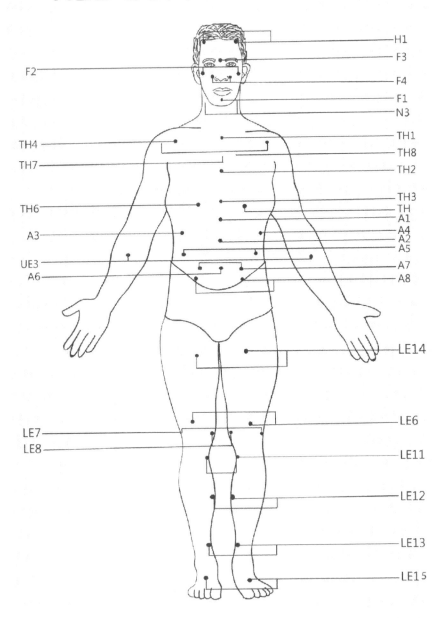

• F2 – deafness, toothache, sore eyes, arthritis.

- F4 – sinusitis, facial paralysis, trigeminal neuralgia, blocked nose
- F1 – mouth ulcers, toothache, facial paralysis, jaw problems
- N3 – dry mouth, mumps, tonsillitis
- TH4 – asthma, cough, bronchitis, pneumonia
- TH1 – pharyngitis, bronchitis, asthma, vocal cord problems, hoarse voice
- TH6 – jaundice, hepatitis, enlarged liver, gallstones
- TH7 – cardiac spasms, heart problems
- TH8 – heart valve problems, cardiac spasm
- TH2 – insufficient lactation, bronchial spasm, chest pain
- A3 – hepatitis, enlarged liver
- TH5 – chest pain, ischemia, cardiac spasm
- TH2 – chest pain, mastitis, bronchial asthma, insufficient lactation
- TH3C – bronchitis, chest pain, bronchial asthma
- F3- rhinitis, vertigo, sinusitis, dizziness
- HI – migraine, facial paralysis, blurred vision, trigeminal neuralgia, eye pressure
- LE15- arthritis
- LE14 – itching of the groins, endometriosis
- LE6 – knee pain, knee cap problems, knee joint, thigh pain
- L13 – liver problems, irregular menstruation, urine incontinence
- A7- irregular menstruation, ovarian dysfunction, appendicitis, infertility
- LE11 – abnormal uterine bleeding, irregular menstruation, wet dreams, dysmenorrhea
- LE12 – irregular menstruation, uterine bleeding, menstrual cramps
- LE13 – liver problems, kidney problems, urinary incontinence, irregular menstruation
- A8 – endometriosis, irregular menstruation, cystitis, hernia
- LE8- uterine bleeding and irregular menstruation
- LE7 – knee cap problems, thigh pain, hip pain, knee pain
- A4- diabetes, enlarged spleen
- A5- kidney stones, constipation, kidney dysfunction, kidney pain
- UE3 – shoulder pain
- A1 – peptic ulcers, gastritis, bloated stomach, vomiting, indigestion, hiccups
- A6- irregular menstruation, appendicitis, vaginal discharge

These cupping points are called **Tibb Cupping Points** and should only be used if you're using the dry cupping technique.

Hijama Cupping Point

Hijama is a cupping technique where blood is drawn out through small skin incisions. It is a technique used by Hippocrates and is practiced in different countries during the ancient times, including Greece, Saudi Arabia, Persia, and Turkey. There are different cupping points in the hijama therapy as illustrated in the next page:

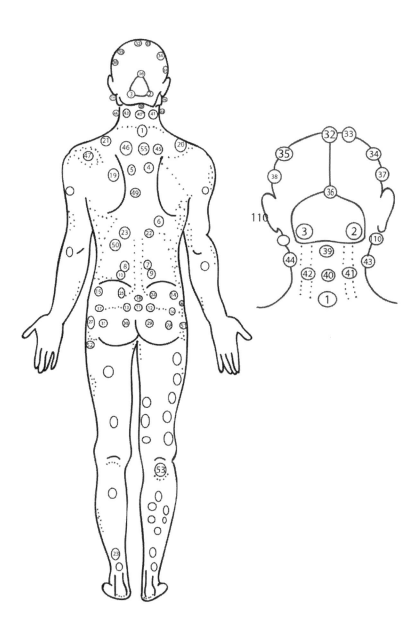

Figure 1.1: Cupping points at the back, including the head

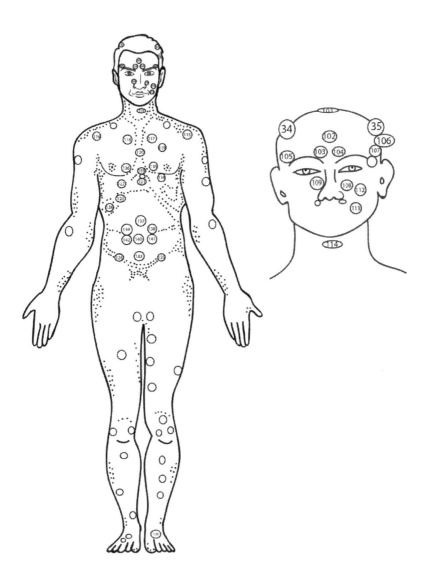

Figure 1.2: Cupping points in the front of the body, including the front of the face.

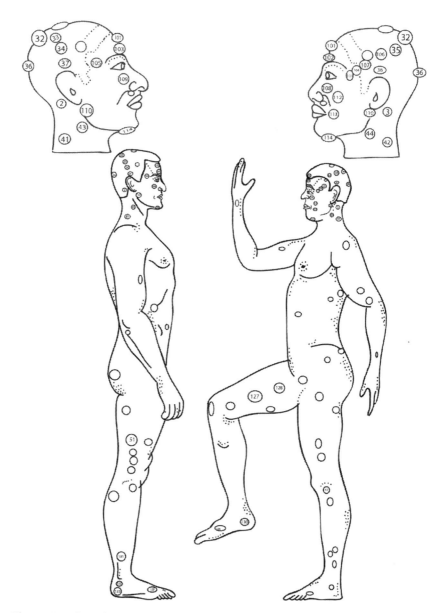

Figure 1.3: Cupping points from the sides of the body including the face
NOTE: You can download a PDF copy of the images on
www.maryconradrn.com. Subscribe to the email list to grab the copy.

Disease	Symptoms	Hijama Cupping Points
Knee pain	Swelling and stiffness, instability, pain, popping or crunching noises, instability, weakness, and redness	13, 12, 11, 1, 55, 54, and 53
Oedema	Puffiness of the tissue under the skin, stretched or shiny skin, weight gain, chest pain, difficulty breathing, bloating	130, 55, 1, 10, and 9
Rheumatism	Fever, anemia, limping, joint deformity, joint tenderness, fatigue, joint pain, joint swelling, fever, tingling, numbness	55, 1, and the part of the body where you experience pain
Right leg sciatic pain	Numbness and pain in the right leg	1,11, 12, 55, 51, 26, and the specific part of the body where you experience pain
Left leg sciatic pain	Numbness and pain in the left leg	11, 1, 13, 52, 27, and the specific part of your leg where you feel discomfort and pain
Cataract	Blurred vision, sensitivity to glare, seeing lights and halos	1, 36, 55, 104, 101, 10, 9, 34, 35, and on your hairline, right above your forehead
Glaucoma	Blurred vision, sudden sight loss, head	36, 55, 1, 104, 101, 10,9, 34, and 34

	pain, severe eye pain, seeing bright lights and rainbow-colored circles	
Diarrhea	Cramps, watery stools, bloating in your belly, nausea, throwing up	139, 138, 137, 140, 142, 125, 126, and 143
Irritable bowel syndrome	Gas, bloating, abdominal pain, cramping, constipation, diarrhea, mucus in the stool	6, 1, 55, 48, 6, 7, 8, 15, 4, 17, 16, 45, 46, and dry cupping on 137
Renal disease	Nausea, fatigue, weakness, sleep problems, decreased mental sharpness, loss of appetite, sleep problems, muscle cramps and twitches	9, 10, 55, 1, 42, 41 and dry cupping on 140, 137
Stomach ulcers	Dull pain in the stomach, heartburn, acid reflux, weight loss, nausea, vomiting	55, 7, 1, 50, 8, 41, 42, and dry cupping on 140, 139, 138, 137
Neck pain	Stiff neck, soreness, sharp or stabbing pain in the neck that radiates down into the fingers and shoulders	55, 1, 20, 21, 40, and the part of your neck where you experience pain
Shoulder pain	Frozen shoulder, instability, rotator cuff disorders, sleep problems, persistent itching, chest pain, sleep problems,	1, 55, 20, 21, 40, 1, and the part of your shoulder where you experience pain

	vomiting, nausea	
Back pain	Aching and dull sensation at the back, stabbing pain that runs from the leg to the foot, inability to move, inability to flex the back	55, 1, and make sure to cup on both sides of your back and spine. You can also place the cup directly to the part where you experience pain.
Gout	Swelling, pain, and tenderness in the big toe joint, itching of the skin around the affected area, red and purplish skin around the affected area	55, 28, 1, 30, 29, 31, 121, and the part where you experience pain
Rheumatoid arthritis	Tender joints, fatigue, stiff joints, joint deformity, fatigue, fever, swollen joints, limping	55, 120, 36, 49, 1, and on the part of your body where you experience pain and swelling
Abdominal pain	Belching, gas, indigestion, heartburn, pelvic discomfort, chest discomfort	55, 7, 8, 1, and dry cupping on 137, 138, 140, 139. You can also cup on both sides of your back.
Hypertension	Severe headache, difficulty breathing, chest pain, vision problems, confusion, fatigue, pounding in your ears and chest	1, 2, 3, 11, 12, 13, 32, 55, 6, 48, 101, 7, 8, 10, and 9
Hemorrhoids	Itching in the buttocks, fecal leakage, irritation around the buttocks, painful bowel movements, blood in stools	121, 55, 1, 6, and dry cupping on 139, 138, 137
Muscle spasm	Muscle pain, lump in the affected area	Dry cupping on the affected area

Tingling arms	Tingling sensation and numbness in the arms, hands, or both	55, 1, 40, 21, 20, affected joints and arm muscles
Tingling feet	Tingling or burning sensation in the feet and hands caused by kidney failure, diabetes, and vitamin deficiency	11, 12, 13, 55, 1, affective muscles, and foot joints
Poor blood circulation	Dry skin, dizziness, vertigo, fatigue, hair loss, numbness, shortness of breath, lack of stamina, skin infection, muscle cramps, foot ulcers, leg ulcers, cold hands and feet, shortness of breath, edema, irregular heartbeats	11, 55, 1, and around 10 cups lined on both sides of the spine.
Weak immune system	Pink eye, sinus infections, yeast infections, pneumonia, diarrhea	49, 120, 55, and 1
Hemiplegia	Weakness and stiffness in the body, difficulty with balance, depression, blurred vision, having a hard time swallowing food, heightened emotional sensitivity, loss of bladder control, poor memory.	13, 12, 11, 35, 34, 1, and the affected area.
Involuntary urination	Involuntary excretion of urine typically used by weakened pelvic floor muscles, diabetes, nerve damage	Dry cupping on 139, 138, 137, 143, 142, 126, and 125
Infertility	Inability to conceive, pain during menstruation, thinning hair, weight gain,	55, 6, 1, 11, 13, 12, 125, 49, 26, 42, and 41

	problems with ejaculation, small and firm testicles, pain in testicles	
Skin diseases		55, 49, 120, 7, 8, 11, 6, 1, and on affected areas of the skin.
Heart disease	Palpitations, dizziness, weakness, faster heartbeat, shortness of breath, sweating, vomiting, dizziness, anxiety, extreme weakness, irregular heartbeats, pounding in your chest, fatigue, fainting, rapid weight gain, limited ability to exercise	55, 19, 119, 1, 46, 47, 134, and 133
Sores	Blister and ulcers on the skin, headache, and sometimes, fever.	120, 129, 55, and 1
Varicose veins	Bleeding from the varicose pain, dark and purple veins, muscle cramps	55, 28, 1, 29, 132, 30, 31 and around the veins. But, do not cup over the veins as this will restrict the blood flow.
Thyroid disease	Fatigue, weight changes, dry skin, muscle weakness, depression, slowed heart rate, impaired memory	42, 41, 55, 1
Migraine	Pain on both signs of your head, mood changes, increased urination, thirst, yawning	1, 2, 3, 106, 55, and the part of your head where you experience pain. You can only do dry cupping on your head area.
Tinnitus	Ringing, buzzing and whistling sounds	1, 20, 21, 42, 41, 114, 49, 44, and 43

Convulsions	Clenching of teeth, grunting, drooling, eye movements, nausea, anxiety, uncontrollable muscle spasms and vertigo. Convulsions are usually caused by head injury, epilepsy, heart disease, drug abuse, low blood sugar, brain tumor, heat intolerance, and high blood pressure.	13, 12, 11, 114, 1, 55, 101, 36, 107, and 101
Neuritis	Flashing lights, pain, loss of color vision, vision loss in one eye, and dizziness.	110, 111, 113, 112, 114, 55, 1 and the affected part of the body.
Vaginal bleeding	Excessive or heavy bleeding, bleeding after sex, and spotting between periods.	Dry cups 55, 3, 1, and under each breast until the bleeding stops.
Menstruation problems	Dysmenorrhea, premenstrual syndrome, skipped periods	137, 139, 140, 143, 142, 138, 125, 126, 55, and 1
Liver disease	Chronic fatigue, loss of appetite, jaundice, itchy skin, chronic fatigue, nausea, and dark urine color. There are many types of liver disease such as hepatitis, alcohol-related liver disease, non-alcoholic fatty liver disease, primary biliary cirrhosis, and haemochromatosis.	55, 1, 48, 42, 41, 122, 51, 123, 124, 6, and 46. You also need to place five cups on the right outer leg.
Gastritis	Abdominal bloating and pain, nausea, indigestion, loss of appetite, hiccups, black stools, and vomiting	55, 1, and 121

	blood	
Depression	Decreased energy, persistent anxious feeling, irritability, insomnia, feelings of hopelessness, suicide attempts, and thoughts of suicide	55, 1, 11, 32, 6, and below the knees.
Chronic constipation	Hard and lumpy tools, swollen belly, few bowel movements, and small tools	11, 55, 1, 12, 13, and 29
Erectile dysfunction	Inability to get an erection, reduced sexual desire, having the problem of keeping an erection	55, 6, 11, 13, and 12
Elephantiasis	Fever, pain above the testicles, pain in testicles, enlarged groin lymph nodes, swollen spleen, swollen liver, white urinary discharge, massively swollen legs	55, 11, 1, 13, 120, 121, and 49
Amenorrhea	Hair loss, milky nipple discharge, headache, pelvic pain, acne, and vision changes	1, 29, 55, 136, and 135
Varicocele	Dull and recurring pain in the scrotum, enlarged veins in the scrotum, and lump in one of the testicles	11, 1, 55, 12, 13, 29, 31, 126, 125

Remember that you should not place the cup on an open wound. Do not place the cup directly on a vein or an artery as this could restrict the movement of the blood.

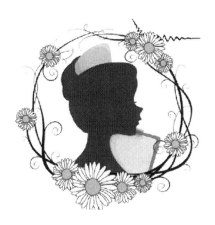

Chapter 7

Cupping and Trigger Points

As mentioned earlier, cupping releases the scar tissue adhesions between the muscle and the fascia, improving your mobility. It also releases trigger points.

A trigger point is an irritable muscle band that attaches the myofascia and the muscle. Trigger points are usually found in the neck, back, and shoulder muscles when these muscles are overused for long periods of time. Trigger points can cause discomfort and real problems for athletes. These points can inhibit motion by keeping the muscles stiff and short. These points produce muscle contraction that can cause nerve entrapment.

Aside from the Tibbs and Hijama cupping points, the cups are also applied directly to the trigger points to ease muscle pain and improve mobility. The suction the cup creates a negative pressure on the affected area, stretching the thickened fascia of the muscles and improving the athlete's movement.

There are several trigger points in the body, including:

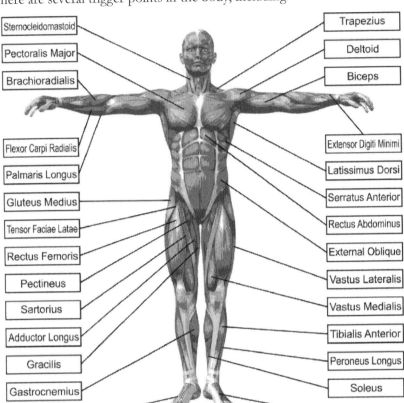

Sternocleidomastoid

Pectoralis Major

Brachioradialis

Flexor Carpi Radialis

Palmaris Longus

Gluteus Medius

Tensor Faciae Latae

Rectus Femoris

Pectineus

Sartorius

Adductor Longus

Gracilis

Gastrocnemius

Extensor Digitorum Brevis

Trapezius

Deltoid

Biceps

Extensor Digiti Minimi

Latissimus Dorsi

Serratus Anterior

Rectus Abdominus

External Oblique

Vastus Lateralis

Vastus Medialis

Tibialis Anterior

Peroneus Longus

Soleus

Extensor Hallucis Brevis

1. **Subclavius** – This is a small triangular muscle located between the first rib and the clavicle.

2. **Pectoralis major**- This is a fan-shaped muscle located in your chest area. It makes up most of your chest muscles.

3. **Pectoralis minor** – This is a thin muscle located in the upper part of your chest and is beneath the pectoralis major.

4. **Sternalis** – This is located in front of the pectoralis major and is parallel to the margin of the sternum.

5. **Anterior deltoid** – This muscle forms the rounded contour of your shoulder. The anterior deltoid is also known as front delts.

6. **Serratus anterior** - This is a saw shaped muscle located in your rib area.

7. **Triceps** – The triceps is a large muscle located on the back of the upper limb. It is responsible for the extension of your elbow joint. In short, it allows you to straighten your arms.

8. **Biceps** – This is a muscle located in your upper arm – between your elbow and shoulder. You use this muscle when you lift things and is frequently used during strength training.

9. **Palmaris longus** – This is a visible spindle-shaped muscle located near your palms and you usually use it to rotate your wrist.

10. **Pronator teres** – The pronator teres is located in the forearm. You use it to turn your forearms so you can see your palms.

11. **External oblique** – The external oblique is located in your abdomen area and it is the largest muscle of the lateral anterior abdomen. It is supplied by the subcostal and thoracoabdominal nerve. It is responsible for the rotation of your torso.

12. **McBurney's point** – This muscle is located at the right side of your abdomen. When this area is tender, it's a sign of acute appendicitis.

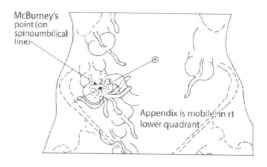

McBurney's point (on spinoumbilical line)

2/3

Appendix is mobile in rt lower quadrant

13. **Adductor longus** – This muscle is located in the thigh and flexes your hip joint and is responsible for the adduction of your hips.

14. **Gracilis** – This is a superficial muscle that's located on the medial

side of your thigh. This muscle medially rotates, adducts, and flexes the hip.

15. **Levator scapulae** – This muscle rotates and elevates your scapula. It is located at the side and back of your neck.

16. **Upper trapezius** – This is one of the two large superficial muscles that extends from the occipital bone to the lower thoracic vertebrae. This rotates, retracts, depress, and elevates the scapula.

17. **Supraspinatus** – This muscle is located at the upper back. At the back of your shoulders and below your neck.

18. **Iliocostalis thoracis** – This muscle is located in your rib area and it is used to extend and flex the vertebral column both unilaterally and bilaterally.

19. **Infraspinatus** – The infraspinatus is a thick triangular muscle that rotates and stabilizes the arm. It is located at the back of your shoulder.

20. **Teres minor** – This is a narrow and elongated muscle located in the rotator cuff. It laterally rotates the arms and stabilizes the humerus.

21. **Rhomboids** – This connects the upper extremity of the vertebral column. It medially rotates and pulls the scapulae.

22. **Lower trapezius** – This is often called as the "bitchy point" by registered chiropractors. It is located at the left side of your back. It adducts and rotates the scapula. Lower trapezius fibers have TrPs or trigger points that cause upper cervical pain. These trigger points can also cause headaches.

23. **Gluteus maximus** – This muscle rotates and extends the hip joint. It also extends the knee and abducts the hips. You use this muscle when performing different exercises such as dead lift, squats, kettlebell swings, quadruped hip extensions, hip thrusts, reverse hyperextension, and glute-ham raise.

24. **Iliopsoas** – This is the combination of two muscles – the iliacus and psoas major. It is located in the abdomen and runs to the thighs. It flexes the hips and is known to be the strongest of all the

hip flexors.

25. **Erector spinae** – The erector spinae consist of three thin and long muscles that runs up each side of the vertebral column. These muscles are called spinalis, longissimus, and iliocostalis.

26. **Gracilis** – The gracilis is a long strap-line muscle that runs from the pubic bone to the side of the knees. It rotates and flexes the leg medially. It also adducts the thigh.

27. **Adductor longus** –This is a skeletal muscle that's located in the thigh. It adducts the thigh and the hip. It also flexes the hip joint. If this muscle is overworked, you'll experience pain, tension, or discomfort in the area.

28. **Sartorius** – The Sartorius muscle is a thin muscle that runs along the thighs. It runs across the anterior and the upper part of the thigh. Its name was derived from the Latin word that literally means tailor. It is also known as a tailor's muscle.

29. **Piriformis** – This muscle is a pear-shaped muscle that's located in the gluteal region of your limb. It is located partly in the pelvis, just above the buttocks area.

30. **Hamstrings** – Hamstrings are muscles located at the back of your thigh. It flexes the knees and extends the hips.

31. **Biceps femoris** – The biceps femoris is located below the hamstrings. It laterally rotates, extends, and flexes the knee joints.

32. **Quadratus lumborum deep** – This is located in your spine area. This trigger point plays a key role in the development of hip pain complications, chronic low back pain, and sciatica symptoms.

33. **Gastrocnemius** – This muscle is located at the back of the lower leg. It is a major muscle in the calf. It is a two-joint muscle and flexes the knees and the foot. Overuse of this muscle can lead to Achilles tendon pain.

34. **Soleus** - This muscle is located in the calf. You use this muscle if you are walking or standing. If the fascia around the soleus thickens, you'll develop the compartment syndrome - a disease that leads to blood clots, neuropathy, and atrophy of muscles

35. **Extensor digitorum longus** – This is a pennate muscle that's located in the front part of your leg, above your feet. This muscle extends the toes.

36. **Vastus medialis** – This is an extensor muscle that's located in the thigh. It extends your knees. When this muscle is stressed or overworked, you'll experience knee pain.

37. **Tibialis anterior** – This muscle is located near the shin and it is responsible for the inversion and the dorsiflexion of the foot. Overusing this muscle can restrict your movement over time.

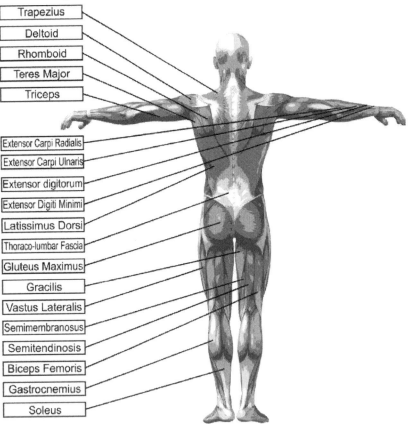

If you experience pain on the trigger points, you can place the cup on them directly. Cupping on the trigger points increases the blood flow in that area, improving the flexibility of the muscle. This improves mobility, which also improves sports performance.

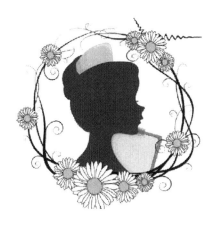

Chapter 8

Acupuncture and Cupping Therapy

Acupuncture is a popular Traditional Chinese Medicine technique in which trained therapists insert thin needles into the skin. It treats various conditions such as muscle spasms, pain, neck pain, osteoarthritis, allergies, depression, and knee pain. Like the cupping therapy, acupuncture improves one's health by improving the flow of blood and qi in the body. Acupuncture and cupping are used together to treat various diseases.

An acupuncture point is the part of the body where you insert the needle. These points were created to correspond to the number of days in a year. Originally, there were 365 acupuncture points. These points were mapped around fourteen acupuncture channel lines. One channel for each of the 12 organs, one along the midline of the stomach, and one channel along the spine. Over time, the number of acupuncture points grew to around 2,000.

Each acupuncture point is associated with a list of diseases that they can treat. These acupuncture points are also used in sports cupping, so it's important to be familiar with these points.

There are fourteen acupuncture channels, namely the heart, large intestine, lungs, pericardium, small intestine, triple heater, gall bladder, kidney, liver, stomach, spleen, urinary bladder, conception vessel, governing vessel, and extra points.

The distance between points is measured in cun, which is the measure of the width of the thumb at the knuckle.

Lungs

LU1 Zhongfu – This is located on your left shoulder and it stops cough and late stage lung diseases. It is measured 6 cun away from the sternum.

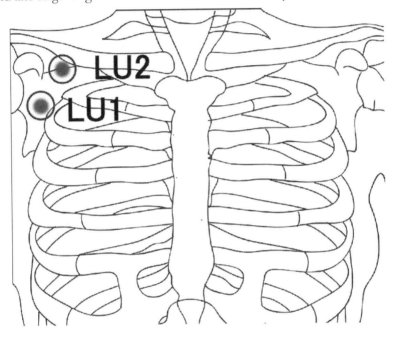

LU2 Yunmen – This is located 1 cun above LU1. It stops cough.

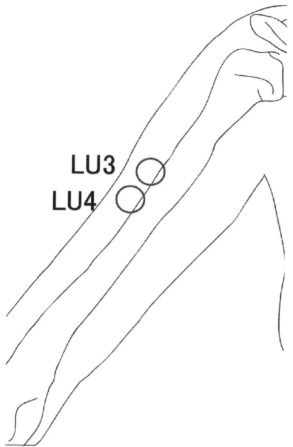

LU3 Tianfu – This regulates the descending and ascending of the life energy qi. When this area is blocked, you'll experience drowsiness, cough, shortness of breath, nosebleed, and goiter.

LU4 Xiabai – This is located on the upper arm and below the armpit. It regulates the qi in the cun difference

LU5 Chize – This is located in the biceps brachi tendon. It clears lung heat and opens the waterways. It also helps remove the phlegm from the lungs.

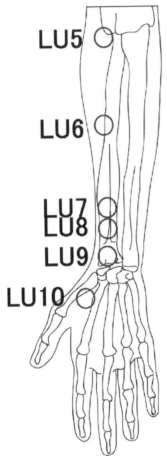

LU6 Kongzui – You can find this acupuncture point above the wrist. It regulates the lung qi.

LU7 Lieque – This is located right above the wrist and it opens the nose and removes phlegm. There's a 0.5 cun distance between LU7 and LU8.

LU8 Jingqu – This is located above the wrist crease and it targets the lungs and throat.

LU9 Taiyuan – This point is located on the side of the radial artery, near the wrist. It is located 1 cun below LU8. There's also a 7 cun distance between LU6 and LU9.

LU10 Yuji – It clears the lung heat and stops the cough. It also calms the mind.

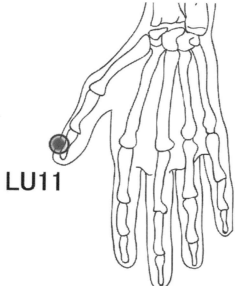

LU11 Shaoshang – It is located in the first thumbnail radial corner. It opens the orifices and it targets the throat.

Large Intestine

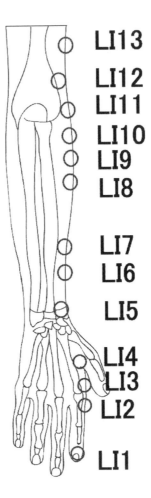

LI1 Shangyang – This is located at the radial side of your index finger. It targets the shoulder and throat. It brightens your eyes and extinguishes inner wind.

LI2 Erjian – This is located on top of LI1.

LI3 Sanjian – This is located on top of LI2.

LI4 Hegu – This is located in between the thumb and index finger. It is located on top of LI3.

LI5 Yangxi – This is located on the wrist.

LI6 Pianli – This acupuncture point is located on top of LI5 with about 3 cun distance between.

LI7 Wenliu – It regulates the intestines. It is located about 5 cun above the wrist.

LI8 Xialian – This is located at four cun below the elbow crease.

LI9 Shanglian – You can find this acupuncture point right above LI8, below the elbow and 1 cun above the LI8.

LI10 Shousanli – This is located right below the elbow, 1 cun from LI9.

LI11 Quchi – This is located at the elbow crease, 2 cun above LI10.

LI12 Zhouliao – This acupuncture point is located above the elbow and it targets the arms. It is located 1 cun from LI11.

LI13 Shouwuli – This is located three cuns above the elbow crease. It removes the phlegm and it relaxes the tendon. It is located 2 cun from LI12.

LI14 Binao – This acupuncture is located at the lower end of the deltoids. It relaxes the tendons and removes the stagnation of the qi. It targets the arms, eyes, and shoulder.

LI15 Jianyu – This is located on top of the shoulder blade. It targets the arms and shoulders.

LI 16 Jugu – This point is located in between the scapular spine and acromion. It disperses lumps and it helps cure duct obstruction syndrome.

LI17 Tianding – This is located at the side of the throat.

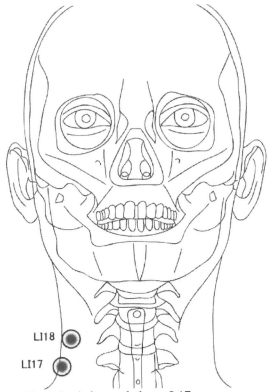

LI18 Futu – This point is located above L17.

LI19 Heliao – This is located between the nose and mouth.

LI20 Yingxiang – This is located beside the nose wing.

Stomach

ST1 Chengqi – This enlightens the eyes and clears the heat in the eye. It targets the mouth, face, and eye. It is located below the eye.

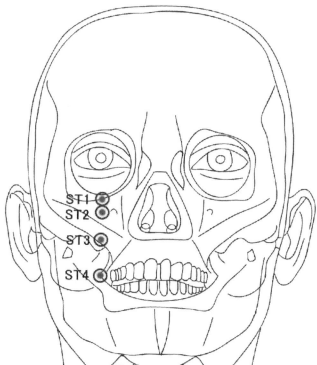

ST2 Sibai – This is located at below ST1.

ST3 Juliao – This point is located below ST2.

ST4 Dicang – This is located on the cheek, below ST3.

ST5 Daying – This is located below St4, below the mouth.

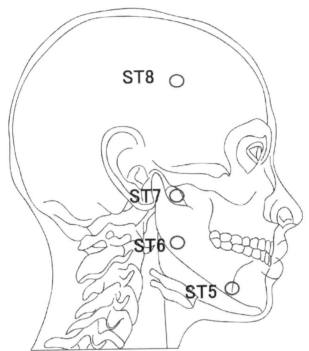

ST6 Jiache – This acupuncture point is located at the side of the mouth.

ST7 Xiaguan – this is located at the side of the face, next to the ear.

ST8 Touwei – This is located in the head, above the ear.

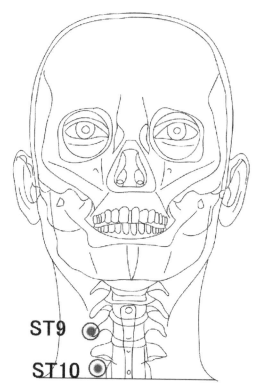

ST9 Renying – This is located in the neck, below the chin.

ST10 Suitu - This is located in between of ST11 and ST8. It regulates the throat qi and expels the wind from the throat.

ST11 Qishe – This is located below the neck, near the shoulder blade. It removes lung heat and phlegm.

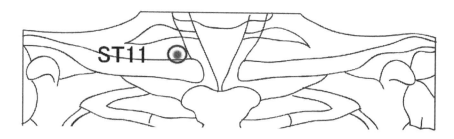

ST12 Quepen – This point is located in the top margin and the middle of the clavicle.

ST13 Qihu – Located below ST12.

ST14 Kufang – Located below ST13.

ST15 Wuyi – This is located below ST14 and within the line that connects the center of the nipple to the clavicle.

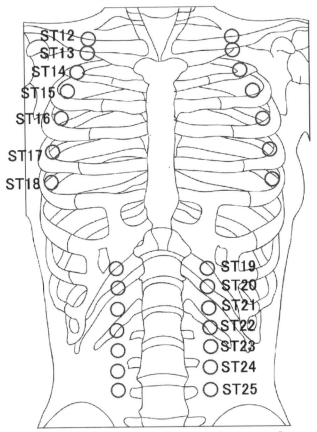

ST16 Yingchuang – This is located in the chest area. It regulates the flow of the qi in the chest.

ST17 Ruzhong – This is located in the breast area.

ST18 Rugen – This point reduces edema and stops cough.

ST19 Burong – This point is located in the rib area below the chest.

ST20 Chengman – This is located below ST19.

ST21 Liangmen – This is located below ST20.

ST22 Guanmen – This is located below ST21.

ST23 Taiyi – This acupuncture point is located below ST22. It regulates the intestines and the stomach. It removes the phlegm and relaxes the mind.

ST24 Huaroumen – This is one cun above the umbilicus. It regulates the stomach and intestines.

ST25 Tianshu – This is located 2 cun lateral to the belly button. It regulates the spleen, stomach, and intestine.

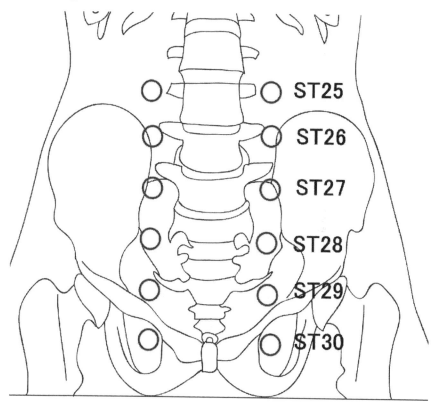

ST26 Wailing – It is located one cun below the navel. It removes the dampness and regulates the stomach.

ST27 Daju – This is located below the navel and it regulates the qi.

ST28 Suidao – This is also located below the navel and below ST27.

ST29 Guilai – It is located 1 cun below ST28.

ST30 Qichong – It is located above the thigh and below ST29.

ST31 Biguan – This removes the duct obstruction and expels wind. This is located in the leg.

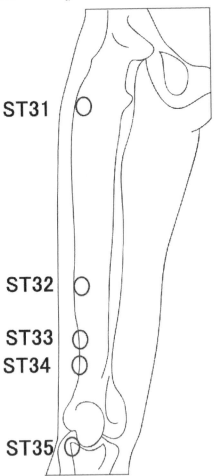

ST32 Futu – This is located about six cun above the knee.

ST33 Yinshi – This is located below ST32 and three cun above the knee.

ST34 Liangqiu – This acupuncture point is two points above the knee.

ST35 Dubi – This is located in the knee and in the cavity, that's lateral to the ligament.

ST36 Zusanli – This is located below the knee and it improves the function of spleen and stomach.

ST37 Shangjuxu – This regulates the intestines and the stomach. It is located below the knee and above three cun below the knee.

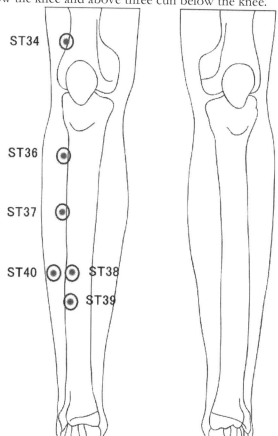

ST38 Tiaokou – This is located below ST37.

ST39 Xiajuxu – This is located below ST38.

ST40 Fenglong – This is located beside the ST38.

ST41 Jiexi – This is located at the midpoint of the crease of the ankle.

ST42 Chongyang – This is located below the ST42.

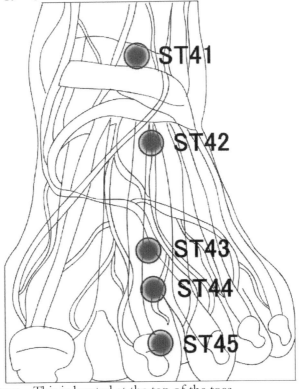

ST43 Xiangu – This is located at the top of the toes.

ST44 Neiting – This is located below ST44.

ST45 Lidui – This is located in the 2nd toe.

Spleen

SP1 Yinbai – This is located on the medial side of your big toe. This point stops bleeding and regulates the spleen.

SP2 Dadu – This is located above SP2 and it regulates the spleen. It clears the mind, too.

SP3 Taibai – This is located above SP2 and near the heel. It strengthens the spleen and regulates the intestines.

SP4 Gongsun – This is located at the side of the feet.

SP5 Shangui - This is located at the base of the metatarsal bone, on top of the feet. It stops the bleeding and it regulates menstruation and intestines.

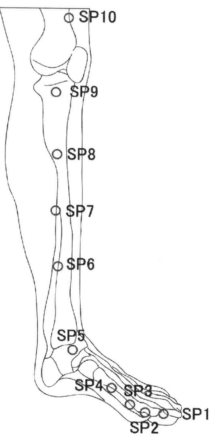

SP6 Sanyinjiao – This is located on the posterior margin of the shin bone. It regulates the liver and the spleen.

SP7 Logu – This is 6 cun above the posterior margin of the shin bone. It targets the leg and the abdomen.

SP8 Diji – This is located three cun below SP9. It harmonizes and cleanses the spleen. It also regulates the uterus.

SP9 Yinlingquan – This is located at the side of the knee. It regulates the spleen and improves the function of the urinary track.

SP10 Xuehai – This is two cun below above the medial border of the patella. It regulates menstruation.

SP11 Jimen – This is located at the back of the thigh.

SP12 Chongmen – This is located at the side of the pelvis area.

SP13 Fushe – You can find this acupuncture point above SP12, at the side of the pelvis area.

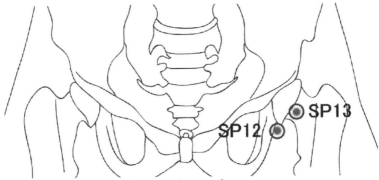

SP14 Fujie- This is located below the navel area.

SP15 Daheng – This is located above SP14.

SP16 Fuai – This is located above SP 15.

SP17 Shidou – This is about 6 cun away from the center of the chest.

SP18 Tianxi – This is directly above SP17.

SP19 Xiongxiang – This acupuncture point is located above SP19.

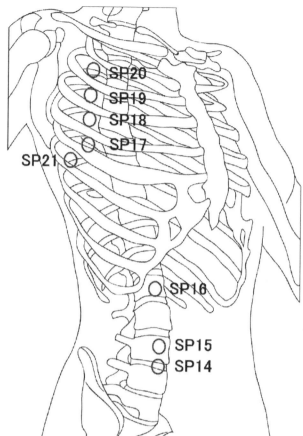

SP20 Zhourung – This is located below the shoulder blade and above SP 19

SP21 Dabao – This is located at the site of the breast.

Heart

HE1 Jiquan – This is located in the armpit.

HE2 Qingling – This point is three cun above the elbow.

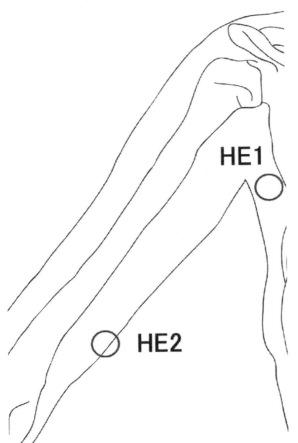

HE3 Shaohai – This is located in the elbow area. It calms the mind and it removes channel obstruction.

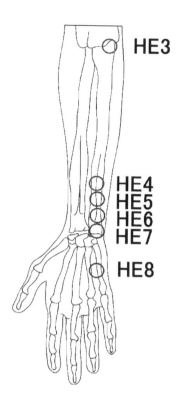

HE4 Lingdao - This is above 1.5 cun above the wrist.

HE5 Tongli – This is directly below HE4.

HE6 Yinxi – This point is below HE6.

HE7 Shenmen – This is directly below HE7.

HE8 Shaofu – This is located in the hand, on top of the pinky finger.

HE9 Shaochong – This is located in the nail area of the pinky finger.

Small Intestine

SI1 Shaoze – This is located at the side of the nail area of the pinky finger.

SI2 Qiangu – This is located above SI1.

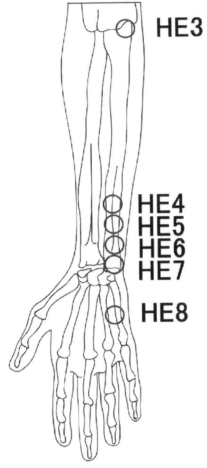

SI3 Houxi – This point is located at the base of the pinky finger.

SI4 Wangu – This is located on the ulnar side of the palm.

SI5 Yanggu – This point is located at the ulnar end of the transverse crease. It clears the heat and it removes the humidity in the knees.

SI6 Yanglao – This is located on the wrist area.

SI7 Zhizheng – This is located between the hand and elbow.

SI8 Xiaohai – This is located at the elbow area. You'll see this acupuncture point when you flex your elbow.

SI9 Jianzhen – This is located on top of the armpit.

SI10 Naoshu – This is located in the shoulder area.

SI11 Tianzhongshu – This point is located right below the shoulder blade.

SI12 Tianchuang – This is located on top the shoulder blades. It targets the scapula, shoulder, and trapezius.

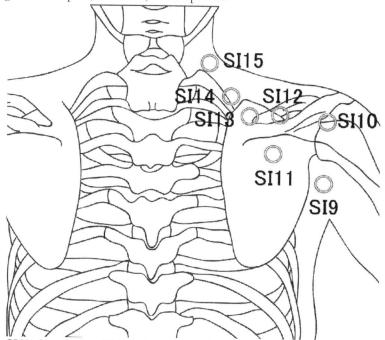

SI13 Quyuan – This is located at the end of the supraspinal cavity of the scapula.

SI14 Jianwaishu – This is located in the levator muscle of the scapula.

SI15 Jianzhongshu – This is located at the side of your neck. Below your ear.

SI16 Tianchung – This is located at the side of the neck.

SI17 Rianrong – This is located in the jaw area. It expels heat and resolve dampness.

SI18 Quanliao – This is located in the cheek.

SI19 Tinggong- This is located near the ear area.

Bladder

BL1 Jingming – This is located in between the eye and the nose.

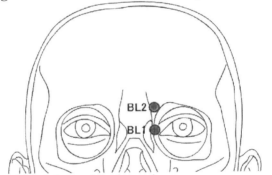

BL2 Zanzhu – This is located in the eyebrow area.

BL3 Meichong – This is located at the center of your scalp.

BL4 Gucha – This is located beside BL4.

BL5 Wuchu – This point is above BL5.

BL6 Chengguang – This is located on top of your head around 1.5 above BL6.

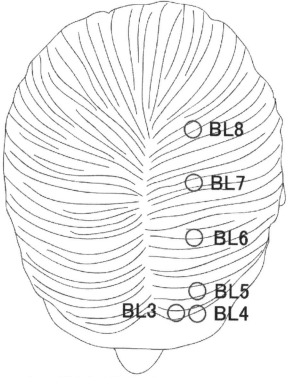

BL7 Tongtian – This is 1.5 cun above BL6.

BL8 Luoque – This is 1.5 cun above BL7.

BL9 Yuzhen – This is located at the back of the head, near the ear.

BL10 Tianzhu - This point is below BL9.

BL11 Dazhu – This is located below the neck, beside the shoulder blade.

BL12 Fengmen – This point is also located below the neck, near the shoulder blade.

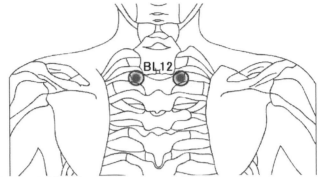

BL13 Feishu – This is located on top of the chest area.

BL14 Jueyinshu – This is located on top of the chest area.

BL15 Xinshu – This is located at the center of the chest area.

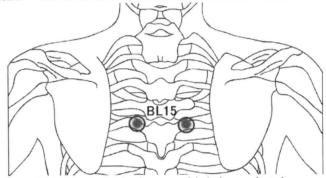

BL16 Dushu – This regulates the heart and it is located at the center of the chest.

BL17 Geshu – This is located at the center of the chest.

BL18 Ganshu – This acupuncture point is leveled with T9. It clears heat and brightens the eyes. It also nourishes the blood.

BL19 Danshu – This point is leveled with T5 and located at the center of the rib area.

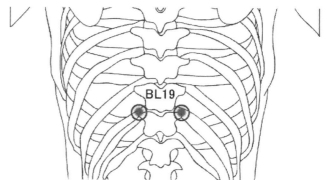

BL20 Pishu – This is leveled with T11 and it is located above the stomach area.

BL21 Weishu – This acupuncture point is located in the stomach area.

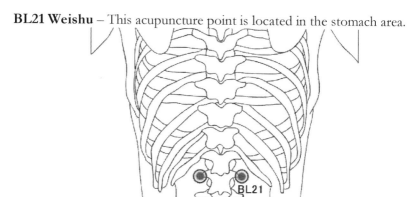

BL22 Sanjiaoshu – This is located in the stomach area. It opens the water way.

BL23 Shenshu – This acupuncture point is located in the stomach area, above the navel.

BL24 Qihaishu – This point is located in the stomach area and it strengthens the lower back. It also regulates menstruation.

BL25 Dachangshu – This is located around 1.5 cun lateral to GV3 and level with L4. It strengthens the lower back and improves the function of the large intestine.

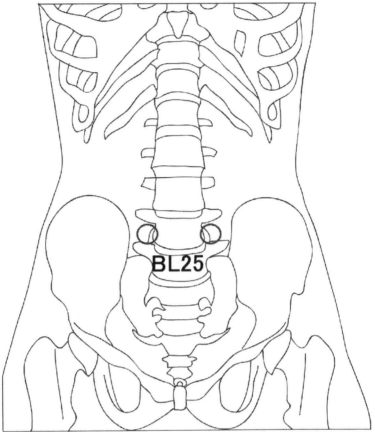

BL26 Guanyuanshu – This point strengthens the lower back and improves the function of the urinary tract.

BL27 Xiaochangshu – This is located in the pelvic area.

BL28 Pangguangshu – This is located directly below BL27.

BL29 Zhonglushu – This acupuncture point is below BL28.

BL30 Baihuanshu – This is located below BL29.

BL31 Shangliao – This is located at the center of the pelvis area and around 1.5 cun lateral to BL27.

BL32 Ciliao – This is directly below BL31.

BL33 Zhongliao – This acupuncture point is below BL32.

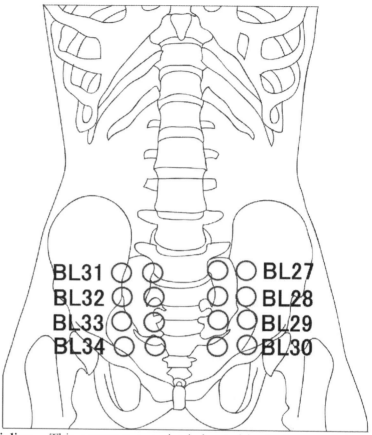

BL34 Xialiao – This acupuncture point is located in the lower pelvis area and below BL33.

BL35 Huiyang- This is located near the tail bone.

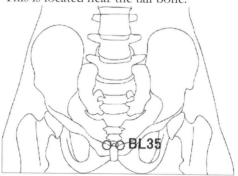

BL36 Chengfu – This is located right below the buttocks.

BL37 Yinmen – This is around 6 cun away from BL36.

BL38 Fuxi – This is located at the back of the knee.

BL39 Weiyang – This acupuncture point is below BL38.
'

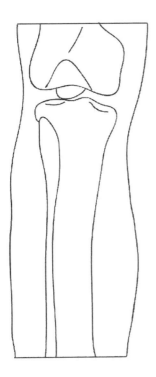 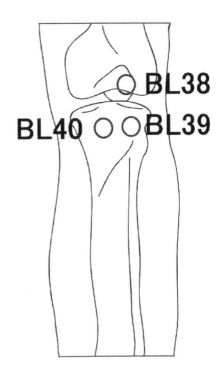

BL40 Weizhong – This is located beside BL40.

BL41 Fufen – This point is 3 cun away from the midline along the spine area.

BL42 Pohu – This is located on the spinal border of the scapula.

BL43 Gaohuangshu – This nourishes the heart and the spleen. It is located at the upper back.

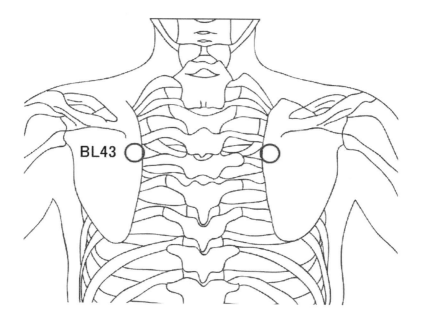

BL44 Shentang – This is located below BL44 and around 3 cun lateral to GV11.

BL45 Yixi – This is located 3 cun away from the midline. It relieves cough and it removes heat.

BL46 Geguan – This is located at the back and it regulates the function of the stomach. It also regulates the middle burner.

BL47 Hunmen – This acupuncture point is located at the back. It regulates the liver qi and it improves the function of the tendon.

BL48 Yanggang – This is three cun away the midline. It removes the heat in the gallbladder.

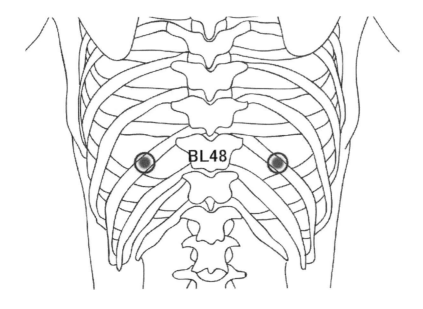

BL49 Yishe – This is located at the back.

BL50 Weicang – This point is 3 cun from the midline. It regulates the qi and relieves pain.

BL51 Huangmen – This is 3 cun away from GV5.

BL52 Zhishi –This is 3 cun lateral to GV4. It improves the urinary tract. It strengthens your willpower and back.

BL53 Baohuang – This is located in the buttocks area. It improves the function of the bladder.

BL54 Zhibian – This is located in the sacral area. It improves the urinary tract and treats hemorrhoids.

BL55 Heyang – This is located 2 cun below the popliteal line center of your calf.

BL56 Chengjin – This is below BL55. It is located in the calf area.

BL57 Chengshan – This is below BL40. It relaxes the tendons and treats hemorrhoids.

BL58 Feiyang – This is located above BL60. It treats the hemorrhoids and strengthens the kidney.

BL59 Fuyang – This is located in the Achilles tendon. It improves the function of the dorsal region.

BL60 Kunlun – This is located on top of the feet and near your Achilles tendon. This point improves movement and strengthens the back.

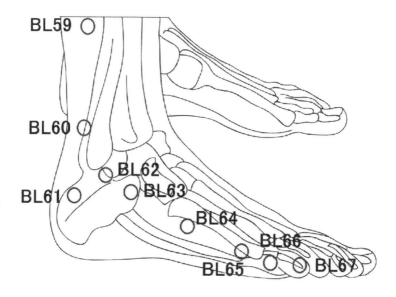

BL61 Pucan – This is around 1.5 cun below the BL60. It relaxes the legs, feet, and muscles.

BL62 Shenmai – This is located at the side of the feet.

BL63 Jinmen- This is located on the lateral side of the foot.

BL64 Jinggu – This is located in your feet.

BL65 Shugu- This is located below BL65.

BL66 Tonggu – This is 1 cun away from BL 65 and located at the base of the pinky toe.

BL67 Zhiyin – This is located in the nail area of the fifth toe (pinky toe).

Kidney

KI1 Yongquan – This is located at the center of the heel.

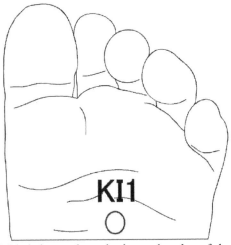

KI2 Rangu – This is located on the lower border of the navicular bone. This is located on top of your heel.

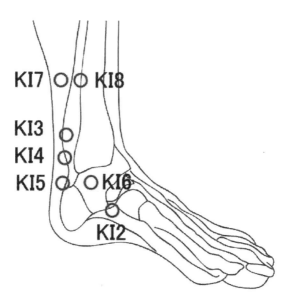

KI3 Taixi – This is located at the attachment of the Achilles tendon.

KI4 Dazhong – This is located below KI3.

KI5 Shuiquan – This is located directly below KI4.

KI6 Zhaohai – This is located in between KI2 and KI5.

KI7 Fuliu – It is located above KI13.

KI8 Jiaoxin – It is located beside KI8.

KI9 Zhubin – This is located in the lower leg, above the feet.

KI10 Yingu – This is on the medial side of the knee.

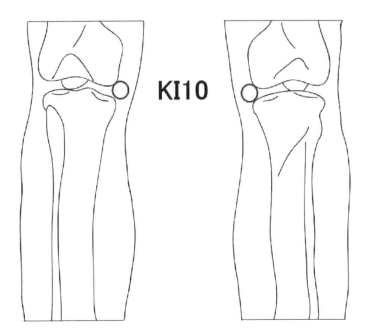

KI11 Henggu – This is located in the pelvis area.

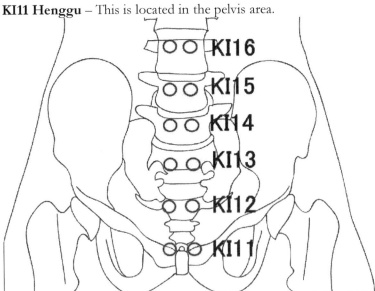

KI12 Dahe – This is located directly above KI11.

KI13 Qixue – This is located 1 cun above K12.

KI14 Siman – This is located 1 cun above KI13.

KI15 Shuiquan – This is located 1 cun above KI14.

KI16 Huangshu – This is located 1 cup above KI15.

KI17 Shangou – This is 2 cun above the navel.

KI18 Shiguan – This is located above KI17.

KI19 Yindu – This is located directly above K18.

KI20 Futonggu – This is located above KI19.

KI21 Youmen – This is located directly above KI21.

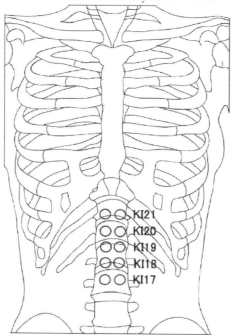

KI22 Bulang – This is located in the breast.

KI23 Shenfeng – This point is directly above 22.

KI24 Lingxu – This point is located directly above KI23.

KI25 Shencang – This acupuncture point is located above KI24.

KI26 Yuzhong – This is located in the shoulder area, above KI25.

KI27 Shufu – This is located on the shoulder area.

Pericardium

PC1 Tianchi – This acupuncture point is located near the nipple. It opens the chest.

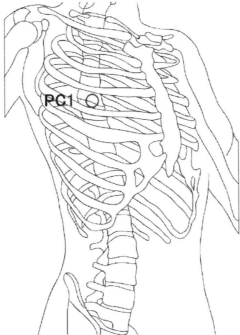

PC2 Tianquan - This is located between the two heads of the biceps. It harmonizes the heart.

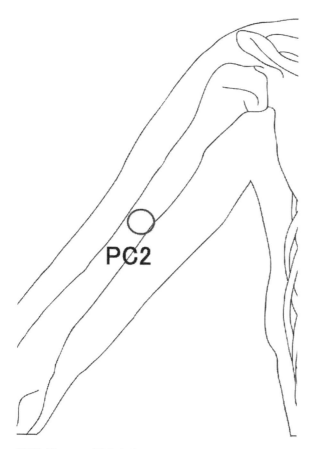

PC3 Quze – This is located on the ulnar side of the biceps. It clears the heat and calms the mind.

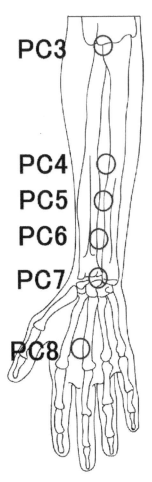

PC4 Ximen – This is five cun above the wrist crease. It invigorates the blood.

PC5 Jianshi – This is three cun above the wrist crease. It is located between the flexor carpi and the palmaris longus.

PC6 Neiguan – This is located 2 cun above the wrist crease. It opens the chest and improves the function of the digestive system.

PC7 Daling – This is located in the middle of the wrist crease.

PC8 Laogong – This is located at the center of the palm.

PC9 Zhongchong – This is located on top of the middle finger.

Triple Burner

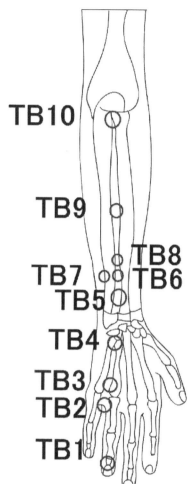

TB1 Guanchong – This is located in the fourth finger.

TB2 Yemen – This is located at the base of the fourth finger.

TB3 Zhongzhu – This is located directly above TB2.

TB4 Yangchi – This is located in the wrist area.

TB5 Waiguan – This is located above TB4.

TB6 Zhigou – This is located above TB5.

TB7 Huizong – This acupuncture point is located beside TB7.

TB8 Sanyangluo – This is located above TB7.

TB9 Sidu – This is located above TB8.

TB10 Tianjing – This is located 5 cun above TB9.

TB11 Qinglengyuan – This is located 2 cun above the elbow.

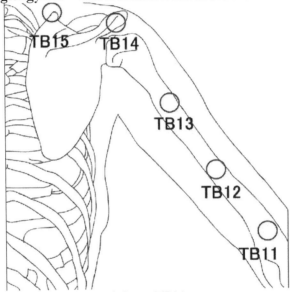

TB12 Xialuo – This is located above TB11.

TB13 Naohui – You can find this acupuncture point above TB12.

TB14 Janliao – This is located in the shoulder area and above TB13.

TB15 Tianliao – This is located in the shoulder blade area.

TB16 Tianyou – This is located at the side of the head.

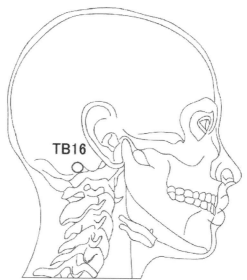

TB17 Yifeng - This is located in the lower part of the ear.

TB18 Chimai – This point is located behind the ear.

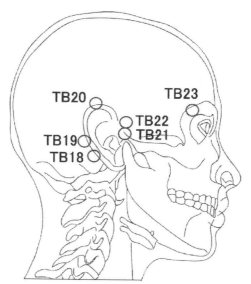

TB19 Luxi – This is located above TB19.

TB20 Jiaosun – This is located on top of the ears.

TB21 Ermen – This is located at the side of the head, near the ear.

TB22 Erheliao – This is located at the side of the head, near the ear. It is directly above TB21.

TB23 Sizhukong - This is located at the end of the eyebrow, near the ear.

Gallbladder

GB1 Tongziliao – This is located beside the eye.

GB2 Tinghui – This point is located at the side of the head, near the ear.

GB3 Shanguan – This is located beside GB2.

GB4 Hanyan – This is located at the side of the head.

GB5 Xuanlu - This is located below GB4.

GB6 Xuanli – This is located below GB5.

GB7 Qubin – This is located below GB6.

GB8 Shuaigu - This is located at the side of the head, above GB7

GB9 Tianchong – This is located beside GB9.

GB10 Fubai - This point is located at the side of the head, behind the ear.

GB11 Touquiaoyin – This is located below GB10.

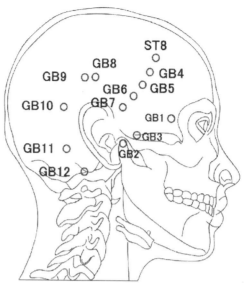

GB12 Wangu – This is located at the side of the head, below the ear.

GB13 Benshen - This is located on top of the hairline.

GB14 Yangbai – This is located on top of the hairline, directly above the eye.

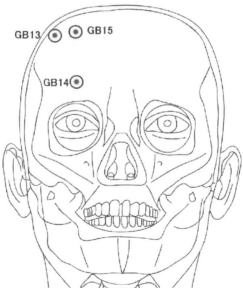

GB15 Linqi -   This is located beside GB13.

GB16 Muchuang – This is located on top of the head.

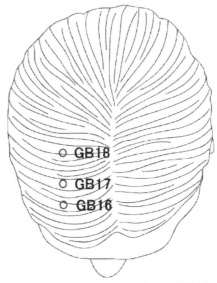

GB17 Zhengying – This is located 1 cun above GB16.

GB18 Chengling – This is located 1.5 cun above GB17. It is located on top of the head.

GB19 Naokong – This is located at the back of the head, 2.25 cun away from GV17.

GB20 Fengchi – This is located at the back of the head, 2.25 cun away from GV16.

GB21 Jianjing – This is located in the middle of the trapezius, in your shoulder area. It improves your mobility and it relaxes the tendons.

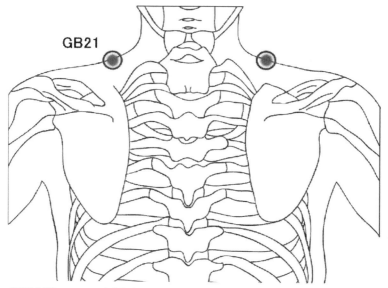

GB22 Yuanye - This is located at the side of the breast.

GB23 Zhejin – This point is located below GB22.

GB24 Riyue – This is located below the breast.

GB25 Jingmen - This is located at the end of the floating rib.

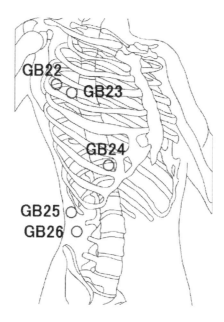

GB26 Daimai – This acupuncture is located below GB25.

GB27 Wushu – This is located in the abdomen area and it regulates the uterus and the girdling vessel.

GB28 Weidao – This acupuncture is located at the side of the stomach.

GB29 Juliao – This point is located at the side of the stomach.

GB30 Huantiao – This point is located in the buttocks area, below GB29.

GB31 Fengshi – Located at the side of the leg, below GB30.

GB32 Zhongdu – This acupuncture point is located at the side of the leg, below GB31.

GB33 Xiyangguan – This acupuncture point is located below GB32.

GB34 Yanglingquan – Like many gall bladder acupuncture points, this point is located at the side of the leg. This is located at the side of the knee.

GB35 Yangjiao – This point is located in the calf, beside GB36.

GB36 Waiqiu – This acupuncture point is right beside GB35.

GB37 Guangming – This acupuncture point is located below GB36.

GB39 Xuanzhong – This is located in the lower leg.

GB40 Qiuxu – This acupuncture is located in the ankle.

GB41 Zulinqi – This point is located near the pinky toe.

GB42 Diwuhui – This acupuncture point is located in the foot, right next to the heads of the fifth and fourth metatarsal.

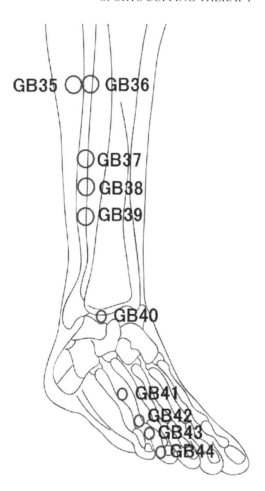

GB43 Xiaxi – This acupuncture point is located between the fifth toe and the fourth toe. It controls the yang energy of the liver and it removes excess body heat and dampness.

GB44 Zuqiaoyin – This is located near the corner of the nail of the 4th toe. It brightens the eyes and controls the yang energy of the liver.

Liver

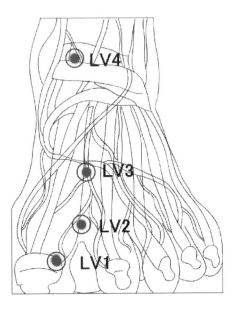

LV1 Dadun – This acupuncture point is located in the lateral side of your big toe. It is around 0.1 cun from the corner of the toenail.

LV2 Xingjian – This point is located between the second and first toe. It controls the liver yang and it extinguishes the inner wind. It calms the mind and it resolves the heat and the dampness of the body.

LV3 Taichong – This is located on the dorsum of the foot, above LV2. It controls the liver yang, calms the mind, and it regulates menstruation. It also resolves spasms.

LV4 Zhongfeng – This is located above LV3, near the ankle.

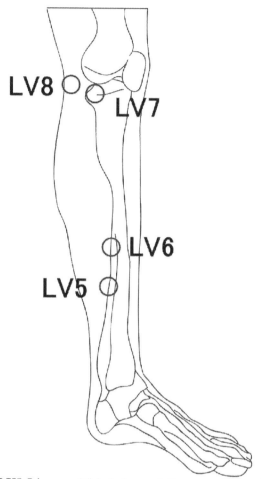

LV5 Ligou – This is located five cun above the ankle. It resolves the dampness and heat in the lower part of your body.

LV6 Zhongdu – This acupuncture point is seven cun above the shinbone. It removes channel obstruction and helps relieve pain in the lower abdomen.

LV7 Xiguan – This is located at the side of the knee and it resolves dampness. It helps resolve knee pain.

LV8 Ququan – This is located at the side of the knee beside LV7.

LV9 Yinbao – This acupuncture point is located four cun above the knee. It regulates the function of the liver.

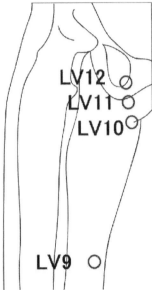

LV10 Zuwuli – This point is located three cun below the pubic area. It relaxes the muscles and tendons. It also eases leg pain.

LV11 Yinlian – This acupuncture point is two cun below the pubic area. It relaxes the muscles and the tendons. It also helps relieve leg pain.

LV12 Jimai – This point is one cun above LV11 and it is situated right beside the pubic region of the body.

LV13 Zhangmen – This point is located on the lateral side of the abdomen below the end of the eleventh rib. It improves the function of the spleen and the liver. It eases rib pain.

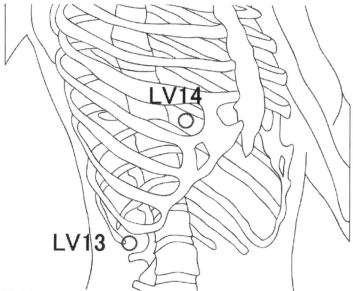

LV14 Qimen - This is located directly below the nipple. It removes the qi stagnation in the liver. It improves the function of the stomach and the liver.

Conception Vessel

CV1 Huiyin – This is located in the middle of the perineum. It regulates the genitals and the orifices (nostrils, ear canals, mouth, anus, vagina, nipple, nasolacrimal ducts).

CV2 Qugu – This is located at the upper margin of the pubic area. It strengthens kidney and improves the function of the reproductive system.

CV3 Zhongji – This is located four cun below the belly button and above CV2. It improves the function of the kidney. It regulates menstruation.

CV4 Guanyuan - This is about 2 cun above the pubic area. This acupuncture point regulates menstruation and it regulates the function of the small intestine.

CV5 Shimen – This is 3 cun above the pubic area. It removes the dampness in the uterus and it regulates the qi in the lower part of the body.

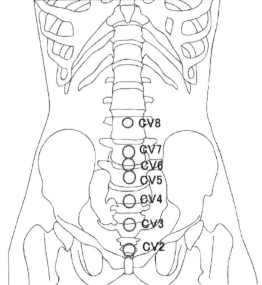

CV6 Qihai – This acupuncture point is 1.5 cun away from the belly button. It targets the genitals, uterus, and lower abdomen.

CV7 Yinjia0 – This is located 1 cun below the belly button. It regulates the function of the uterus and menstruation.

CV8 Shenque – This is located at the belly button. This acupuncture point strengthens the spleen.

CV9 Shuifen – This is about 1 cun away from the belly button.

CV10 Xiawan – Located two cun above the belly button.

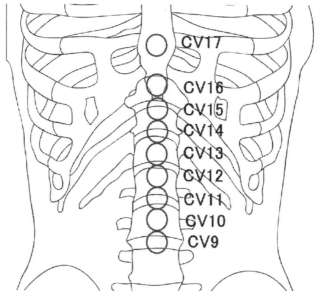

CV11 Jianli – Located three cun above CV8 (the belly button).

CV12 Zhongwan – This acupuncture point is located directly above CV11.

CV13 Shangwan – This point is directly above CV12.

CV14 Juque – This is located above CV13.

CV15 Jiuwei – This point is located seven cun above the belly button. It opens the chest and relieves mental issues such as obsession, palpation, fear, and manic-depressive disorder.

CV16 Zhongting – This is located right below the breasts.

CV17 Tanzhong – This is located in between the nipples. It opens the chest.

CV18 Yutang – This is located at the middle of the chest.

CV19 Zigong – This acupuncture point is located directly above CV18.

CV20 Huagai – This acupuncture point is located above CV19 and below the neck.

CV21 Xuanji – This acupuncture point is located in between the shoulder blades.

CV22 Tiantu – This is located in the neck area.

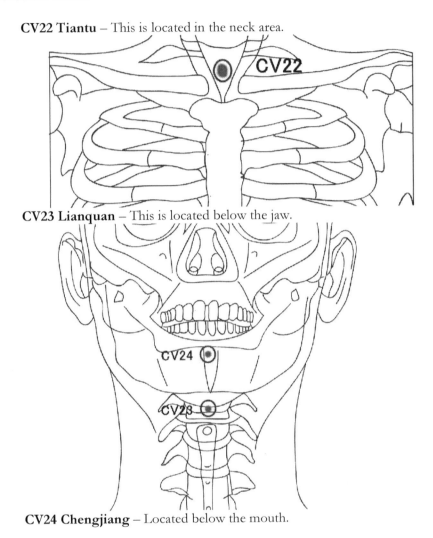

CV23 Lianquan – This is located below the jaw.

CV24 Chengjiang – Located below the mouth.

Governing Vessel

GV1 Changqiang – This point is located between the anus and the coccyx. This point helps treat epilepsy, manic-depression, and hemorrhoids.

GV2 Yaoshu – This is located in the anus area and it strengthens the lower back.

GV3 Yaoyangguan – This is located L4. It strengthens the legs and lower back.

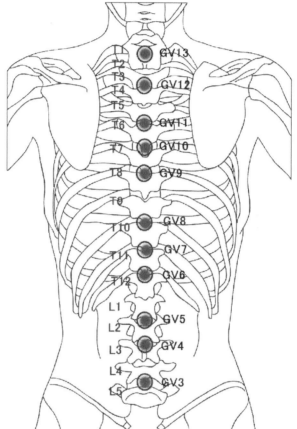

GV4 Mingmen – This is located at the back, in between L3 and L4.

GV5 Xuanshu – This acupuncture point is located at the lower back, right above GV4.

GV6 Jizhong- This is located at the back, beneath T11. It improves the function of the spleen and it removes internal wind.

GV7 Zhongshu – This point strengthens the spine and the spleen.

GV8 Jinsuo – This point is located below T9 and it relaxes the tendons.

GV9 Zhiyang – This acupuncture point is below in the upper back. It regulates the gallbladder and liver. It opens the chest.

GV10 Lingtai – This point is located in the upper back above GV9. It helps remove toxic heat.

GV11 Shendao – This is located at the back, right below the neck. It helps remove the lung heat.

GV12 Shenzhu – This is located on the midline, at the upper back. It lightens the lung heat and removes internal wind.

GV13 Taodao – This acupuncture point is located at the back, below the neck.

GV14 Dazhui – This is located at the back part of the neck. It helps ease fatigue.

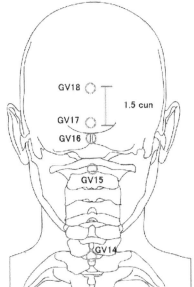

GV15 Yamen – This is located at the back of the head.

GV16 Fengfu – This point is located on the midline of the head.

GV17 Naohu – This acupuncture point is located above the head and it extinguishes the inner wind.

GV18 Qiangjian – This is located directly above G17, on the midline of the head. It calms the mind and removes internal wind.

GV19 Houding – This is located on the midline of the head.

GV20 Baihui – This acupuncture point is located above the head, in between the ears.

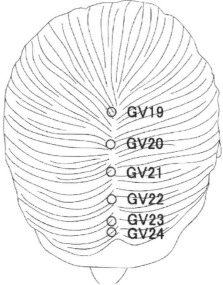

GV21 Qianding – This acupuncture point is located on top of the head and above GV20.

GV22 Xinhui – This is located 1.5 cun above GV21 and it helps minimize mental agitation and stress that athletes often experience.

GV23 Shangxing – This is located in the midline of the head. It opens the nose and lightens the eyes.

GV24 Shenting – This is located right above the hairline and along the midline of the head.

GV25 Suliao – This acupuncture point is located at the tip of the nose. It relieves rhinitis.

GV26 Renzhong – This is located between the lower lip and the nose.

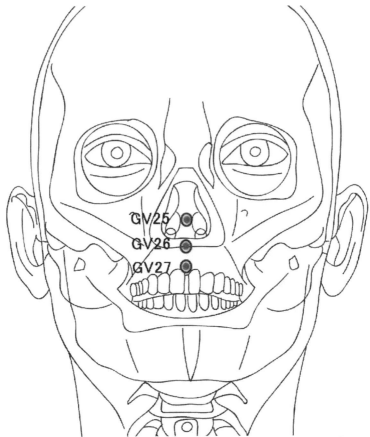

GV27 Diuduan – This is located at the upper edge of the upper lip.

GV28 Yianjiao – This is located on the gums.

Extra

EX1 Sishencong – Sishencong has four points located at the top of the head. It is one cun away from GV20.

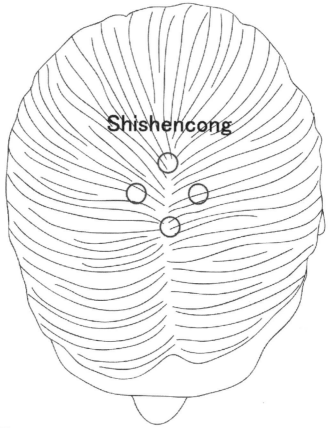

EX2 Yintang – This is located in between your eyebrows. It extinguishes inner wind and it calms the mind.

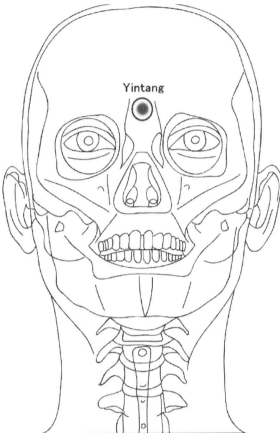

EX3 Taiyang – This acupuncture point is located at the end of the eyebrow. It controls the function of the liver and it improves your eyesight.

EX4 Yuyao – This is located on the middle of the eyebrows. It controls the function of the liver.

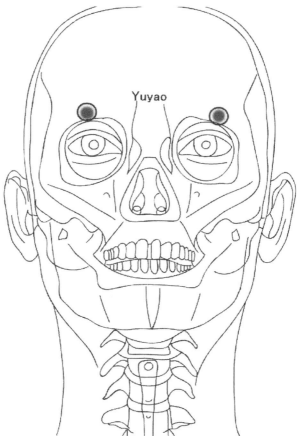

Yuyao

EX5 Bitong – This acupuncture point is located at the side of the nose. It opens the nose and treats rhinitis.

EX6 Jingzhong – This is located on the hip area beside CV6.

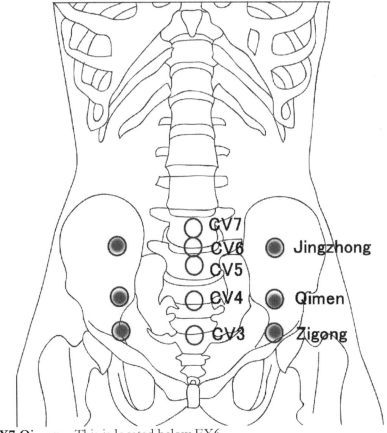

EX7 Qimen – This is located below EX6.

EX8 Zigong – This is located on the sacral area.

EX9 Tituo – This is located 4 cun lateral to CV4.

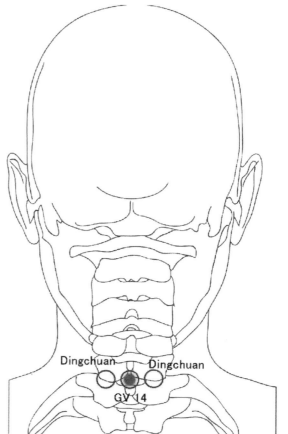

EX10 Dingchuan – Dingchuan is located at the back of the neck and beside GV14. It improves the function of the lungs and reduces breathlessness.

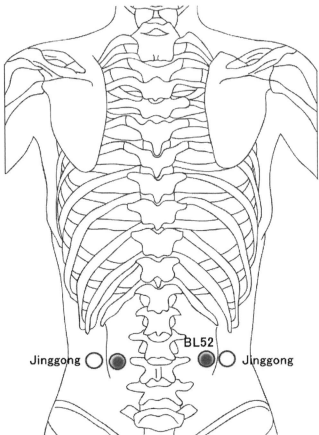

EX11 Jinggong – This is located at the side of the stomach and beside BL52.

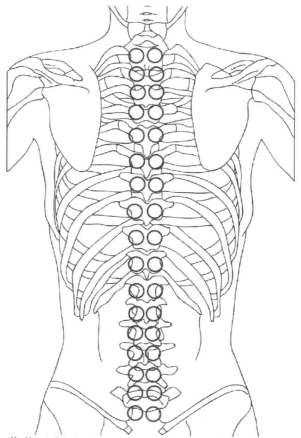

EX12 Huatuojiaji – This is located around 0.5 cun from the spine. This acupuncture point strengthens the back column.

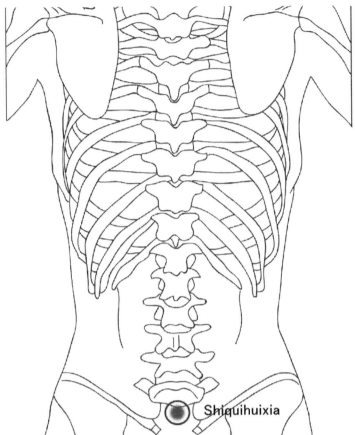

EX13 Shiquihuixia – This is located at the base of the spine and it strengthens the lower back.

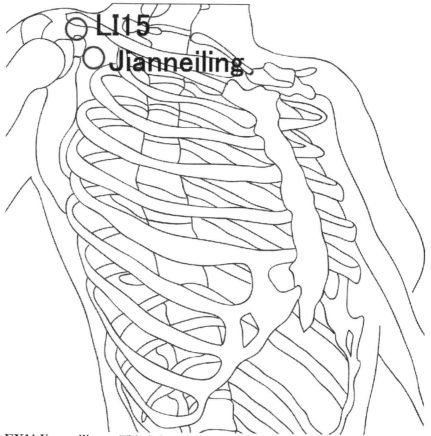

EX14 Jianneiling – This is located near the armpits and below LI15.

EX15 Baxie – This is located in the five webbed fingers. It relaxes the tendons of the wrist, fingers, and hands.

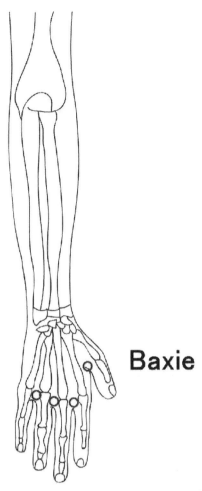

Baxie

EX16 Shixuan – This is located at the tip of the finger.

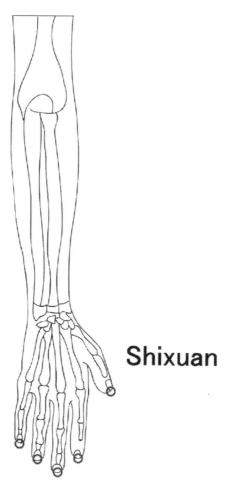

Shixuan

EX17 Xiyan – This is located in the knee. It expels the wind.

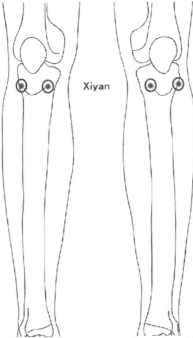

Xiyan

EX18 Dannangxue – This is located at the side of the knee and it is susceptible to pain.

EX19 Laweixue – This is located at the front of the lower leg, in between ST36 and ST37.

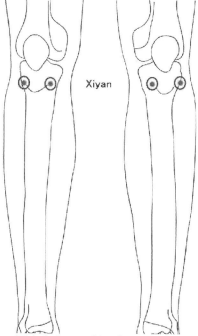

Xiyan

EX20 Bafeng – This is located in the webbing of the toes. It relaxes the tendons and it reduces the spasms and stiffness in the foot.

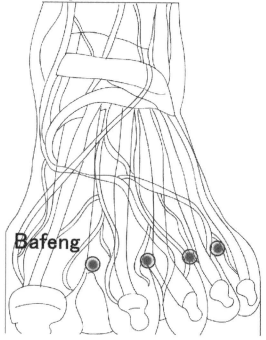

Bafeng

EX21 Erjian – This is located at the back of the ear.

EX22 Anmian – This is located at the navel area.

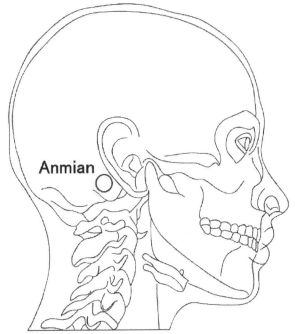

EX23 Qipang – This acupuncture point is located above the wrist.

EX24 Erbai – This is located at the center of the hand. It treats neck pain.

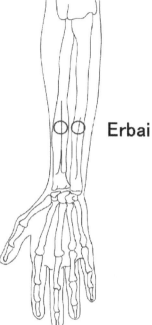

Erbai

EX25 Luozhen – This is located at the center of the hand, in between the middle finger and the index finger.

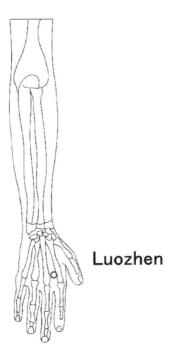

Luozhen

EX26 Yaotongxue – Yaotongxue is comprised of two points located in between the fifth finger and the fourth finger and in between the index finger and the middle finger. These points help treat lower back pain and improve mobility.

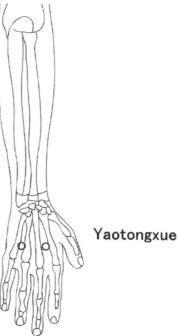

Yaotongxue

EX27 Heding – This point is located above the knee and treats knee injuries.

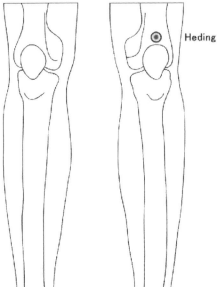

Heding

EX28 Neimadian – This is located on the medial side of the lower leg. It treats leg pain and pain after surgery.

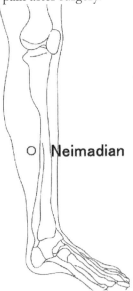

Neimadian

EX29 Naoqing – This is located just above the ankle. It treats mental confusion and improves cognitive function.

For some sports injuries, you'd need to use the acupuncture points in doing the cupping treatment. But, in some cases, you can simply use the trigger points.

MARY CONRAD

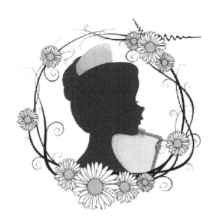

Chapter 9

Common Sports Injuries and How To Use Sports Cupping to Treat Them

Sporting injuries not only affect your performance, but can also have an extremely detrimental effect on your health. Some sporting injuries come with intense psychological effects.

Here's a list of the most common sporting injuries and how to use cupping therapy to treat them.

Ankle Injuries

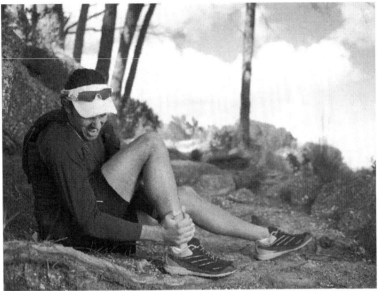

Many athletes use sports cupping for ankle sprains. Ankle injury is painful and it can affect movement. The swelling and bruising associated with ankle injury can also result to sprain.

Football players, surfers, snowboarders, triathletes, rugby players, karate players, and cricket players are susceptible to ankle injuries. To treat this medical condition, you can use medium to strong cupping method in the injured area after the swelling has receded. You can also apply a cup on various acupuncture points such as: SP5 Shangqui, BL60 Kunlun, BL62 Shenmai, K8 Jiaoxin, and K3 Taixi. You can also apply the Hijama cupping method on BL-62 and ST-41 Jiexi.

Achilles Tendonitis

The Achilles tendon is the firm band of tissue that connects the heel bone to the calf muscles. It is also known as the calcaneal tendon. It allows you to walk and helps you stand on tiptoe. It is the strongest and largest tendon in the body and lies directly beneath the skin. It does not have any protective covering so it is prone to inflammation and injury.

Achilles tendonitis affects squash, basketball players, triathletes, divers, professional dancers, rugby players, and football players. It is caused by overtraining, sudden increase in the intensity of the workout, extra bone growth, and tight calf muscles. This disorder is characterized by stiffness and pain along the Achilles tendon. If you have this disorder, you'll feel pain and swelling in your feet after exercising. Achilles tendonitis is one of the most common sports injury. In fact, it accounts five to ten percent of athletic injuries.

To treat this condition, do the moving cupping (massage cupping) technique on the Achilles tendon, starting from the acupuncture point BL57 Chengjin to the calcaneus. Make sure that you get a clearance from your physician prior to attempting this treatment.

Achilles Tendon Rupture

This is the complete tear of the Achilles tendon. This affects rugby players, jumpers, runners, cyclists, gymnasts, football players, volleyball players, and tennis players. Athletes who suffer from this disorder feel a sharp pain in the Achilles tendon. Cupping is not advised.

Medial Tibial Stress Syndrome

The medial tibial stress syndrome is an injury in the front of the outer leg. It is commonly known as Shin Splints. This disorder is caused by repetitive trauma to the connective muscle tissues that surrounds the shin bone (tibia). Weak core muscles, inflexible and tight lower leg, and muscle imbalance can increase the risk of the development of this disorder.

Shin splints affects athletes in sports that involve running and endurance running. It affects squash players, tennis players, football players, triathletes, runners, gymnasts, basketball players, and volleyball players.

To treat this disorder, apply moving cupping therapy to the outer part of the shin bone. Place the cup on ST36 Zusanli and then move it all the way to ST39 Xiajuxu. Do this twice a week for at least two weeks.

Knee Injury

The knee is the heaviest and biggest joint. It is enclosed in a fluid –filled sac called the synovial capsule. It connects the lower leg to the upper leg. Trauma and overuse of the leg can cause knee injury. This condition affects runners, volleyball players, basketball players, rugby players, high jumpers, swimmers, golfers, and martial artists.

To treat knee injury, do medium cupping to ST35 Dubi, GB34 Yanglingquan, Liv8 Quguan, Heiding Extra, and ST34 Liangqui. You can also do Hijama cupping on the site of the injury.

Iliotibial Band Syndrome

This is one of the most common overuse injuries among athletes. It is characterized by aching and pain on the lateral side of the hip and knee. It is usually caused by friction between the hip bone and iliotibial band. Athletes suffering from this disorder feel sharp and burning sensation in the knee and hip.

The iliotibial band syndrome affects runners, cyclists, triathletes, football players, tennis players, weightlifters, and squash players.

To treat this, do medium and strong cupping method on the lateral side of the knee. You can also move the cup to the tensor fascia. You can also apply a cup on the GB30 Huantiao.

Hamstring Injuries

Hamstring injuries can restrict movement and are slow to heal. Athletes with hamstring injuries are recommended to rest for a few weeks.

This injury affects football, rugby, and cricket players. To treat this, you have to do moving cupping from BL36 Chengfu to BL 40 Weizhong. If the pain originates from the lumber spine, you also need to cup DU3 Yaoyanogguan, BL28 Pangguangshu, and BL26 Guanyuanshu.

Quadriceps Femoris Injuries

The quads or quadriceps femoris is located at the front of the thigh. It has four parts – vastus medialis, vastus lateralis, vastus intermedius, and rectus femoris. This injury affects many athletes, especially football and rugby players.

To treat this condition, apply light and medium cupping technique to the external part of your quads (vastus lateralis) and then, move to the front of the quadriceps femoris (rectus femoris).

Hip and Groin Pain

This area accommodates several vital organs such as the small intestine, ureter, cecum, the ascending colon of the large intestine, fallopian tubes, and ovary. If you experience pain in this area, you should take it seriously. It also hosts many tendons, ligaments, veins, arteries, bony structures, and nerves. The hip and groin area also carries a lot of your weight when you are doing household chores and sporting activities.

The hip is basically the ball and socket joint that attaches the pelvis to the femur attaches. A wide array of activities such as running, walking, and jumping affect the hip. Inappropriate footwear and feebleness of the lower back muscles can lead to hip pain. Most types of hip pain is caused by trauma when doing contact sports such as fractures, contusions, tendon or ligament injuries.

Golf, basketball, and football players are susceptible to hip and groin pain because they twist their body often.

To address hip pain, apply the medium cupping method on lower back points, namely BL-53 Baohuang, BL-28 Pannguangshu, and GB-30 Huantiao.

To treat groin pain, use the moving cupping method starting from BL 28 Pangguangshu and then move the cup towards GB28.

Buttock Pain

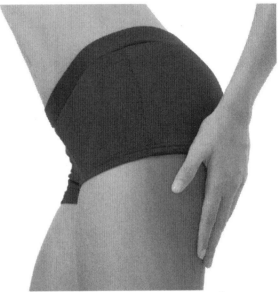

Athletes involved in sprinting and kicking sports often experience buttock pain. This pain may be isolated in the buttock area or it may be associated with posterior thigh pain or lower back pain. This pain is usually caused by problems in the sacroiliac joint, the lumbar spine, and the hamstring attachments on the bony parts of the butt called ischial tuberosities. But, in some cases, buttock pain is caused by more serious health conditions such as ankylosing spondylitis, spondyloarthropathies, psoriatic arthritis, Reiter's syndrome, malignancy, and arthritis associated with inflammatory bowel disease.

Buttock pain can restrict your movement and can negatively affect your performance. To treat localized buttock pain (meaning, you only feel pain in the buttock area), apply medium to strong cupping method on EM-Yaoyan, BL54 Zhibian, GB30 Huantiao, and BL28 Pangguangshu.

If you also feel pain in your legs or lower back, do the moving cupping therapy method following the path of your gluteus maximus muscle.

Lower Back Injuries

Lower back pain is one of the most common medical complaints among athletes and the general population. Most athletes experience lower back pain because of the strain or tightness of the lower back muscles.

Strained or tight lower back muscle leads to spasm, restricting the blood supply in the muscle tissue. This can restrict movement and negatively affect your athletic performance. There are many factors that cause lower back pain, including:

- Twisting the spine while lifting
- Lifting a heavy object
- Poor posture
- Overuse of the lumbar spine

Repetitive swinging motions required for tennis, basketball, cricket, squash, golf, and racquetball can lead to the inflammation and injury of the ligaments, vertebrae, and spinal discs. Spinal stress fractures acquired during contact sports can leave you in constant pain and can restrict your mobility.

Golfers, runners, and tennis players are prone to lower back injuries. If the pain is isolated in the lower back, apply cupping therapy to GV3 Yaoyangguan, BL28 Pangguangshu, and BL26 Guanyuanshu.

If the lower back pain is in the lower back, but radiating towards the buttocks, you should place the cups on GV3 Yaoyangguan, BL54 Zhibian, and BL53 Baohuang. Use light to medium cupping. Allow the cups to sit on the skin for fifteen minutes.

If your back is stiff, you can do the moving cupping therapy following the path of the affected muscle. For example, when treating the stiff erector spinae muscle, your cupping movement should trace the path of the muscle. This means that you should move the cup in vertical motion. You'd need to do the therapy once or twice a week for five weeks. It usually takes ten to twenty cupping therapy sessions to treat lower back injuries.

Shoulder Injuries

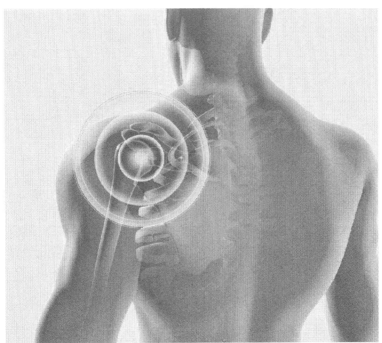

Shoulder injury is the second most common complaint amongst athletes, next to back injury. The shoulder is one of the most challenging body parts to treat. The shoulder is a complex joint that's connected by ligaments and strap like muscle called "rotator cuffs". The shoulder is made of three bones, namely the clavicle, the scapula, and the humerus. It is also made of four joints, namely:

- ➢ *GH (Glenohumeral) Joint* – This is the ball and socket joint that connects the upper arm (humerus) and the scapula (shoulder blade).
- ➢ SC (Sternoclavicular) Joint – This is the joint between the clavicle and the sternum.
- ➢ AC (Acromioclavicular) Joint – This is between the clavicle (collarbone) and the highest part of the shoulder blade called acromion.
- ➢ ST (Scapulothoracic) Joint – This is the joint in between the rib cage and the scapula.

Athletes involved in throwing sports such as baseball, rugby, hockey, golf, tennis, volleyball, and Australian football are susceptible to shoulder injuries. Gymnasts, weight lifters, cyclists, swimmers, and shot-putters also suffer from this type of injury from time to time. Forty percent of the athletes who suffer from shoulder-related injury experience AC joint injuries.

Here are the most common types of shoulder injuries:

Adhesive Capsulitis or Frozen Shoulder

Active athletes are not susceptible to this injury. But, it is a serious condition that affects older athletes. Frozen shoulder is caused by the inflammation or overuse of the GH joint. It is also caused by various diseases such as breast surgery, trauma, diabetes, and hypothyroidism. If you suffer from this condition, your shoulder movement is limited and painful.

Acromioclavicular Joint Arthrosis or AC Joint Degeneration

This is caused by the excessive use of the AC joint. When you have this disorder, you will experience pain in the front part of your shoulder. This pain may spread to the arm, neck, or chest.

Rotator Cuff Injuries

Rotator cuffs are small but strong muscles surrounding the shoulder. There are four types of rotator cuffs namely, the subscapularis, teres minor, infraspinatus, and supraspinatus. The teres minor and the infraspinatus muscles are external rotators. The subscapularis is the internal rotator of the glenohumeral (GH) joint. If you lift your arms up too often, you are susceptible to rotator cuff injuries.

To treat shoulder injuries, you need to use four pieces of size number 2 or number 3 cups. Apply medium cupping method on the TCM (traditional Chinese medicine) points close to the shoulder joint, namely LU2 Yunmen, SI9 Jianzhen, SP20 Zhouron, SI10 Naoshu, SI11 Tianzhong, SJ14 Jianliao, and LI16 Jugu. If you can also feel pain in the arm, add LI14Binao, LI15 Jianyu, and SJ13 Naohui. If you can also feel pain in the neck, you can add cups on SI12 Bingfeng and SJ15 Tianlao. SJ15 is located between GB21 Jianjing and SI13 Quyuan. Let the cups sit for ten minutes to 20 minutes, depending on the severity of the injury.

You can use the moving cupping therapy on most types of shoulder injuries. But, avoid using this method on dislocated shoulder injuries. Follow the path of the shoulder muscles when moving the cup. It is also best to combine acupuncture and cupping therapy in treating shoulder injuries.

Underperformance Syndrome

All training can lead to occasional loss of energy and performance. This is called the Underperformance Syndrome. According to an issue of the Sports Injury Bulletin published in 2002, UUPS or Unexplained Underperformance Syndrome is a history of fatigue and loss of performance without a medical cause and despite 2 weeks of rest. This condition was defined in 1999 by a group of researchers at Oxford University. This condition affects two percent to ten percent of elite endurance athletes. Fatigue is the number one symptom of this syndrome.

But, in the world of competitive sports, most coaches increase the intensity of the training when the athlete is underperforming. This worsens the fatigue and the underperformance.

Before you use the cupping therapy as treatment for this syndrome, you must use the tongue diagnostic technique of the traditional Chinese medicine to correctly determine the underlying factors that caused the underperformance syndrome. To do this, look at the patient's tongue and examine the color.

Color	Indications
Pale	Pale – blood or qi deficiency Pale, thin, and dry – blood deficiency Pale and wet – qi deficiency Pale and swollen – qi deficiency Pale, swollen, and wet – yang deficiency
Pink	Normal or just mild disorder
Red	Red – excessive body heat Red and yellow coat – excess heat in the body Red and wet – damp heat Dry and red – injuries
Dark Red	Extreme body heat
Purple	Stagnation Purple and place - cold
Blue	Severe internal cold

If the underperformance is caused by blood or qi stagnation, you need to place an empty cup in the middle of the chest for ten minutes daily.

Blood Injury

This sounds funny. How is the blood injured? Blood is a fluid that's transformed from the essence of the food and water that you take and it is produced through the activity of the qi. It circulates in the body and nourishes the body tissue. It contains qi or energy. The qi moves wherever the blood moves. Blood injury happens when your body is overworked or if you have a poor diet. Blood injury is also caused by other factors such as excessive sexual activity, long lasting bleeding, and intense exercise regimen. When your blood is injured, you'll experience dizziness, insomnia, palpitations, aching bones, and muscles. You may also have a hard time

145

breathing and you'll experience profuse sweating.

To treat qi and blood stagnation, blood circulation needs to be increased. You can do this by placing a cup at the front of the chest for about 15 minutes a day. You can also place a cup on LU1 Zhongfu and LU2 Yunmen and the entire back.

Forearm and Elbow Injuries

Athletes are susceptible to elbow and forearm injuries that affect the muscles, joints, bony parts, ligaments, nerves, and tendons. It is caused by overtraining or on-field collision. If the injury is caused by on-field collision, do not use cupping therapy. The patient must be taken to the hospital immediately. You can only use cupping therapy for elbow and forearm injuries that are caused by overuse or overtraining.

Athletes that are involved in golf, swimming, racquet sports, basketball, baseball, bowling, water skiing, weightlifting, gymnastics, rock climbing, and kayaking are more susceptible to forearm and elbow injury.

To treat elbow and forearm injuries, apply either static or moving cupping therapy on the affected area.

Remember that cupping therapy for common sporting injuries should be conducted by certified therapists.

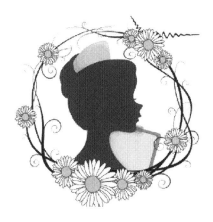

Chapter 10

All You Need To Know About The Bruises

The suction created by the cups will most likely leave a mark on the skin. But, do not worry, these marks are just temporary.

But, there's one thing that you need to know about the marks. The color and the texture of the cup marks can tell a lot about the status of your health.

Bright Red Cupping Marks

This indicates that there is excessive heat in the area and that there's possible inflammation. When this happens, it's helpful to use the flash cupping technique as the skin may bleed. You have to use cooling balms on the marks. But, do not use ice.

Purple Blue

When the skin is purple blue during cupping, it means that there's stagnation. It means that wind is stuck in that area and unable to move. This is called "lamig" in the Philippines. You can use heat therapy to disperse the wind in the area. If there's stagnation in one part of your body, it's best to cup that area often.

Dark Blue to Purple Black

If the skin is dark blue to purple black, it means that there's toxic build up in this area. It also means that there's "poison wind" in that area. The blood in that area of your body is toxic and it needs to be drained.

Pale Whitish

If the skin is pale white during cupping, it means that there's not enough blood circulation in that area because of energy blockage. If this happens, stop cupping immediately and apply a hot compress or heating balm in the area.

Deep Red to Magenta

This means that there's stagnant heat in the area. The skin may be bleeding. After cupping, you may use a trauma liniment. This can help cool and soothe the skin.

Dark Gray

If the skin is dark gray after the cup is removed, this means that the toxins are sinking back into the body. You need to draw out these toxins by cupping that area again or using by using balms.

If the cupping marks do not disappear after two weeks, you need to see a therapist. You may also need to consult a dermatologist if you experience severe skin damage.

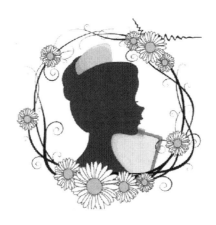

Chapter 11

Frequently Asked Questions About Cupping

Here's a list of frequently asked questions about cupping therapy.

1. Is cupping safe?

Yes. All methods contained in this book are safe and effective when practiced by a trained professional.

2. Can I do this therapy on myself?

Yes, you can do cupping on the frontal aspect of your body. But, if you're not trained, it's best to hire a professional. Doing this on your own might not yield the results you want, especially for specific illnesses, but it can be effective in terms of relaxation.

3. Should I expect marks after cupping?

Yes, marks are often inevitable. But, these marks will fade away between two days to a week at most. The length of recovery often depends on the intensity of the treatment and how long the cups were left on the skin.

4. Does it hurt?

Most often than not, it doesn't. You'll just feel a pulling sensation. But, in some cases, strong cupping may cause pain, which is a sign that the pressure should be elevated to more tolerable levels.

5. Does cupping cause skin damage?

Not at all. The marks that you'll see after cupping are just temporary. The reddish marks are signs that there's an increased blood flow in that area of your body.

6. Can I cup on my face?

Yes, you can but you can only use the light cupping technique on your face. You also need to use smaller cups (cup no. 4, 5, and 6)

7. Can I cup on my private parts?

No, it may cause problems.

8. Will I feel tired after the cupping session?

Yes, you'll most likely feel a little weak after the cupping session. But, some people feel energized right after the cupping therapy. It generally depends on the intensity of the treatment.

9. Does cupping therapy have side effects?

Yes. Aside from the temporary marks on your skin, you might also feel intense hunger after the therapy. You may experience night sweats, vivid dreams, headaches, nausea, and chills. You may even have strong body odor because of the detox.

10. How many times do I have to undergo cupping therapy before I can see the effect?

It depends. But, you can already see improvements after one to two cupping therapy sessions.

11. Can you use cupping therapy on cancer patients?

Yes, you can. It's an effective pain management tool for cancer patients.

However, energy levels as well as overall health status of the patient must be taken into account before doing the session. During the metastatic stage or the last stages of cancer, cupping is contraindicated.

12. Where do I go to get cupping therapy?

You can visit TCM (traditional Chinese medicine) clinics. A lot of sports coaches, Olympic trainers, and physical therapist also do cupping therapy.

13. Can you use cupping therapy as a complementary treatment?

Yes. You can use cupping therapy while undergoing traditional medical treatment. But, if you're taking high doses of medicine, it's best to discuss your plan to undergo cupping therapy with your physician.

14. Can I do cupping therapy when I have a fever?

No. Do not try cupping therapy if you have a high fever or if you are extremely excited.

15. Is it safe to go through cupping therapy on an empty stomach?

Do not try cupping therapy when you're hungry to prevent fainting and severe weakness. Try to eat a little bit before doing the therapy.

16. Is cupping therapy safe for children and old people?

Generally, yes. But, you can only use light cupping method and you have to do it with extreme care.

17. Why do I see bruises?

The suction created by the cup draws up stagnant, old, and non-circulating blood from the area, bringing them up to the surface of the skin. This can leave marks called 'sha'.

18. How long is each session?

Most therapists do massage, too, so one session could last 30 minutes to an hour. The cupping itself can be between 10 to 15 minutes for initial sessions.

19. What do I do after the treatment?

You have to drink a lot of water to flush out all the toxins that were drawn out. Make sure to get plenty of rest after the treatment, do not do heavy physical activities. Athletes and celebrities have no qualms about showing off their cupping marks. But, to avoid infection, make sure that all the marks are covered. It's also important to avoid alcoholic drinks on the day of the treatment.

20. Is it expensive?

Many people think that cupping therapy is expensive since it's the latest celebrity fad, but it's relatively affordable. As of 2017, each session costs around $40 to $80.

Sports cupping is not as popular as the traditional therapy, but several studies show that it can significantly improve sports performance. No wonder, sports superstars like Michael Phelps believe in it.

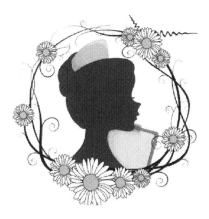

Conclusion

Sports cupping is a relatively new practice that incorporates the old methods of traditional cupping with the newer concepts physical therapy. At present, different physical therapy clinics have slowly adapted the use of cupping for athletes as a way of increasing the rate of recovery and easing post-workout pain. To maximize the effect of using this technique in sports, professionals are qualified to assist you. However, for those who like to do this at home, it can also be quite effective in relieving muscle issues. It would be safer to have a partner when doing this at home.

I hope this book helped you in getting more information on sports cupping and its general benefits. Whether you opt to perform your cupping at home or get certified training, cupping is both a fascinating topic to learn and quite easy to apply with the right level of knowledge.

Finally, if you enjoyed this book, then I'd like to ask you for a favor. Would you be kind enough to leave a review for this book on Amazon? It'd be greatly appreciated!

Follow me on Facebook (Mary Conrad) and Twitter (@authormconrad).

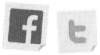

Subscribe to my newsletter to get updates on my latest book and free giveaways!

www.maryconradrn.com

If you have any suggestions or specific natural remedies that you want to have researched and written about, shoot me an email at authormaryconrad@gmail.com. I'm always on the lookout for great new topics to write about. :)

Thank you for taking this journey with me, and good luck!

CHECK OUT MY OTHER BOOKS:

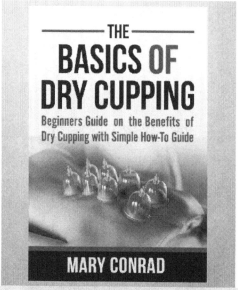

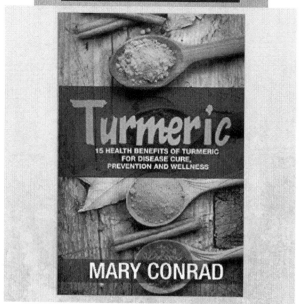

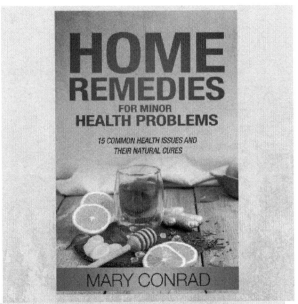

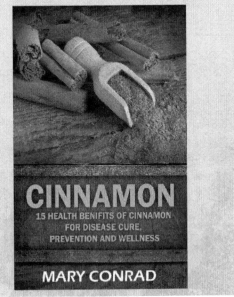

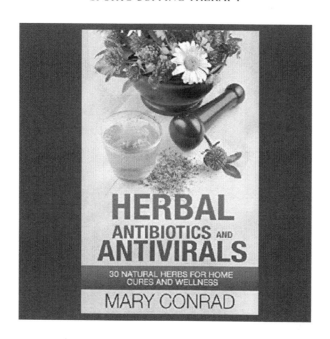

MARY CONRAD

Author Biography

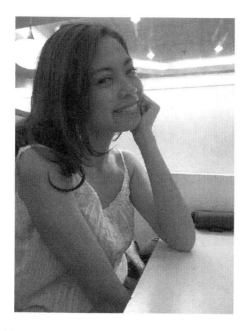

Mary Conrad is a Registered Nurse, who has a strong interest in natural remedies. As a mother, she believes in a holistic approach to health and well-being. Even though she graduated in the health profession, which usually advocates pharmaceutical medication, she believes that prevention is the best step towards health. Backed with scientific research, she wrote these books for both personal information and for others who share the same passion for holistic wellness. It's all about knowing the best natural ways to prevent disease and remedy current health problems. Like every health care provider, she believes in doing no harm, and promoting health. Take a step towards health, and towards nature.

MARY CONRAD